THE
SMART
GIRL'S
GUIDE
TO
POLYAMORY

THE SMART GIRL'S GUIDE TO POLYAMORY

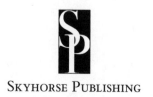

**Everything You Need to Know
About Open Relationships,
Non-Monogamy, and
Alternative Love**

DEDEKER WINSTON

SKYHORSE PUBLISHING

Skyhorse Publishing books may be purchased in bulk at special discounts for sales promotion, corporate gifts, fund-raising, or educational purposes. Special editions can also be created to specifications. For details, contact the Special Sales Department, Skyhorse Publishing, 307 West 36th Street, 11th Floor, New York, NY 10018 or info@skyhorsepublishing.com.

Skyhorse® and Skyhorse Publishing® are registered trademarks of Skyhorse Publishing, Inc.®, a Delaware corporation.

Visit our website at www.skyhorsepublishing.com.

10 9 8 7 6 5 4

Library of Congress Cataloging-in-Publication Data

Names: Winston, Dedeker, author.
Title: The smart girl's guide to polyamory : everything you need to know about open relationships, non-monogamy, and alternative love / Dedeker Winston.
Description: New York : Skyhorse Publishing, 2017. | Includes index.
Identifiers: LCCN 2016050121 | ISBN 9781510712089 (paperback)
Subjects: LCSH: Non-monogamous relationships. | Interpersonal relations. | Marriage. | BISAC: FAMILY & RELATIONSHIPS / Marriage. | FAMILY & RELATIONSHIPS / Love & Romance.
Classification: LCC HQ980 .W56 2017 | DDC 306.8--dc23
LC record available at https://lccn.loc.gov/2016050121

Cover design by Jane Sheppard

Print ISBN: 978-1-5107-1208-9
Ebook ISBN: 978-1-5107-1209-6

Printed in the United States of America

For Emily

Contents

Acknowledgments

My deepest appreciation goes to every person who removed obstacles and helped forge the path ahead. Special thanks to . . .

My agents, Uwe and Brent, for sharing my vision and stroking my ego at all the right moments.

My editor, Nicole, for endless patience for all of my newb questions.

Alex, for making me smile.

My community of friends at The Church, for carrying and supporting me.

Mali, for challenging me to do things right.

My family, for unconditional love.

Jase, for giving me absolutely everything, without reservation, expectation, or obligation, even when I didn't deserve it.

Preface

It was with great trepidation that I started writing a book on poly- amory specifically for women. Though I was raised by a strong, independent single woman, I resisted the label of "capital-F feminist" for so long. From what I saw growing up, feminists were ridiculed. They had so many important things to say about intersectionality, beauty standards, and centuries of oppression, but these opinions were often invalidated by the grossly distorted social caricature of what a feminist was—man-hating, picketing, bra-burning grumps out to ruin everyone's fun. In my formative years, I wanted to speak up against these things, but I feared being stereotyped in the same way.

I was in a stage production of *The Vagina Monologues* during my sophomore year of college. Me, the theater arts major and therefore only "real" actor in the production, saddled with twenty women's studies majors who were full of heart, passion, and spit, but who couldn't vocally project to save their lives. As most of the group took up rehearsal time organizing next week's Take Back the Night rally and discussing the situation in Darfur, I sat in the corner memorizing my lines and hoping the performance wouldn't be too much of a train wreck to invite my theater professors. I couldn't see the forest of feminist liberation for the trees of good presentation.

Humanism. That's what I clung to. My investment in the value and shared plight of all human beings allowed me to wave the banner for equality and stick it to the man without having to get lumped into the "angry feminist" image that I so feared. I recognized the crushing weight of gender inequality, but I rallied for all human beings to have their rights recognized. Our cultural obsession with the differences between the genders was what was holding us back. A rising tide lifts all boats, after all, and everyone would benefit if we could just start focusing on the similarities between human beings rather than the disparities.

This is a philosophy that I hold to this day, particularly in my view of polyamory. Polyamory resonated so strongly with me because I perceived it to be equal-opportunity. It allowed for the recognition that all human beings want love, sex, attention, support, and community. In the world of polyamory, it wasn't strange that I, a woman, wanted a variety of sexual partners with no desire for exclusivity (qualities normally attributed to men). It wasn't strange for a woman to be the primary breadwinner while her romantic partners preferred to be at home. Gender roles were fluid and frequently turned upside down, and everyone involved aimed for equal access to partners, sex, support, and love.

I didn't recognize it initially, but this falls in line with feminist thought. And like feminism itself, my choice to pursue polyamory has been met with all-too-familiar backlash. *Women don't want sex as much as men do. Polyamory will never work, because all women eventually want to settle down with a husband and kids. Women who have multiple partners just have unresolved father issues.* While criticism of polyamorous men can be just as vitriolic, my years spent in this lifestyle have illuminated how cruel society can be to women who color outside the lines, especially when it comes to love, sex, and gender identity.

My journey into polyamory has not been easy or comfortable, but the rewards have been innumerable. All of the highs, lows, and wrong turns have been an intense education about myself—what makes me tick, what sets me off, what turns me on, and what truly brings me happiness. I have found the power to craft relationships that fulfill and energize, and I have discovered more love, security, affection, trust, and stability than ever before. Even though I and countless others have found the same satisfaction, non-monogamous women are still viewed as deviant, attention-seeking, "slutty," or mentally ill. Old-school cultural opinions on female romantic conduct are not congruent with the polyamorous models of equality, honesty, and sex positivity.

These old opinions have infiltrated our movies, TV shows, books, and magazines. Girls are learning these traditional ideas about love and sex from the same places that teach them what kind of exercises to do to get a twenty-four-inch waist and which lip shade to buy that will inspire him to ask them to the prom. The disempowering pop culture of womanhood dictates not only how our bodies should look, but how our hearts should feel.

Without even realizing it, I have found myself facing a feminist issue point-blank, despite all of my years of resistance. My small contribution is to provide a source of relationship knowledge that is empowering and enlivening. This book is an alternative education in love, because for so long there have been so few alternatives that women can turn to. Regardless of whether a woman chooses a romantic life that is monogamous, polyamorous, or somewhere in between, I envision a world where that choice is well-informed, supported, and accepted.

I memorized my lines from *The Vagina Monologues* so well that I still remember them to this day, but to those twenty women's studies majors who wasted valuable rehearsal time for the sake of bettering the world: you had the right idea.

Course Syllabus: An Introduction to Alternative Love

What is love? What does it mean to be in a relationship? These are painfully cliché questions, but human beings have been trying to come up with a satisfactory answer for centuries. No one has been able to agree on a common definition yet, but as a result of all our trying we have a veritable cornucopia of definitions of love. They're all over the movies—*Love means never having to say you're sorry.* They're in every song on the radio—*Love is like oxygen. Love is a battlefield. Baby, don't hurt me, don't hurt me no more.* Go to a church service, and you'll probably hear about it—*Love is patient, love is kind. It does not envy, it does not boast.* Social psychologist Barbara Fredrickson came up with this analytical, yet thorough description:

> *Love is an interpersonally situated experience marked by*
> *momentary increases in shared positive emotions, biobehavioral*
> *synchrony, and mutual care, which, over time, builds embodied rapport,*
> *social bonds, and commitment.*[1]

This definition doesn't make for great song lyrics.

So maybe we can't all get on the same page, but we can all agree that love is some *thing* that is part of the human experience. Call it a feeling, an emotional sensation, a mind-set, a verb, a way of being, but whatever it is, we do know that it *is*. Which leads to the follow-up question, one that is probably the source of more anxiety, confusion, agony, and puzzlement than the original cliché question.

What do we do about it?

This is the face that has launched a thousand ships. There are innumerable books, advice columns, workshops, seminars, dating websites, therapists, and counselors, none of which would exist without countless human beings feeling stumped by that question.

I love this person . . .

But the sex isn't good anymore.

But I'm attracted to someone else.

But my family doesn't like her.

But I want to have kids and he doesn't.

But I am also in love with three other people.

But she doesn't make enough money.

But I still love my ex.

But I don't want to get hurt.

But he doesn't love me back.

What do I *do*?

Love, as much as it delights and intoxicates us, also sends us crashing into the depths of despair and sleepless nights. Solving the ubiquitous "problems" of love is the recurring theme of our soap operas and rom-coms. It keeps us running to the dating books and relationship professionals, seeking some logical, left-brained solution for our irrational, right-brained romantic turmoil.

But as a result of consistently puzzling over this paradox, we are bombarded on a daily basis by those who would give us the holy grail of relationship advice. The secret is to act like a lady, think like a man. Or maybe the key is to accept the fact that he's just not that into you. There might be some value to be found in saving sex for marriage. Or wait . . . perhaps you just need to follow these ten steps to get your man to settle down.

Though the trials and tribulations of love seem to be universal, the solutions, advice, and quick-fixes found in trending Internet articles and on the magazine rack are definitely not. Women in particular are fed a one-size-fits-all script. You want to get married. You want to have babies. You want to lose weight. You want to look pretty. But the script ignores the stark truth that there is very little you can objectively claim that every woman wants. Not every woman is aiming to get married. Not every woman dreams of getting a guy to settle down. Not every woman believes in a soulmate. Not every woman wants to look like a woman. Not every woman is happy with the status quo of long-term monogamy.

That's where this book comes in. Sorry to say, it does not contain all the answers about how to love, who to love, or what to do about it all. What it does provide is a glimpse into a world outside the status quo. Instead of telling you the "rules" about relationships, this book presents the notion of having agency and power when creating relationships. There is no one way it has to be. There is a choice. You don't have to get married. You don't have to stay single to protect your heart. You don't have to have 2.5 kids. You can have ten. Or none. You can roll around on the floor of a swinger's club with someone you just met. You can bring your girlfriend *and* your boyfriend home for Christmas.

If this is your first time picking up a book about polyamory, congratulations—but don't get too excited. If non-monogamy intrigues you as an option for your life, the journey of discovery that you're about to go on is not going to be easy and will be far from comfortable. The further you conceptually pull away from the cultural norms of monogamy and traditional marriage, the more important it will be to self-examine. You will be asking tough questions about what you really want out of your love life and how you want it to look, discovering how you genuinely function as a sexual being, uncovering your deepest desires, defense mechanisms, and motivations. And while the path to self-awareness and personal growth is typically riddled with embarrassing landmarks (your author has made more than a few humiliating mistakes), the best part is that it unlocks the freedom to unapologetically pursue what you want.

The most powerful way to use *The Smart Girl's Guide to Polyamory* is to approach this book with your own life in mind. Make note of what you are drawn to and what you would want to make possible for your love life, as well as what turns you off or scares you. Be aware of thoughts and feelings, positive or negative, that arise as reactions to what you're reading. It can be useful to keep a journal, especially for the personal exploration exercises. You may find much that surprises you about yourself, and you may be even more surprised to see your thoughts and feelings change over time.

Whether you're a seasoned graduate, a timid freshman, or somewhere in between, you'll learn how to discover and craft unique relationships that are healthy, happy, sexy, and tailor-made for *you*. No relationship book can give you the exact answer you need at any given time, but if you're armed with a little advice and a lot of self-knowledge, this book can be an excellent road map for any romantic journey you choose to take.

The Women in This Book

This book would not be possible without the generosity of all of the women who were willing to tell the stories of their nontraditional lives. The women

I interviewed for this book are from all walks of life—young, old, straight, gay, queer, asexual, and transgender. These women represent multiple countries, cultures, colors, and religions. The majority of these women come from Western cultures, though during the writing of this book I was in the midst of traveling through many non-Western countries and compiling information and interviews with non-monogamous women. That research will likely be the subject of another book.

The women in this book shared themselves with me fully, opened up about their most painful and vulnerable moments, and delighted me with their success stories. I sought to tell a story of women and polyamory that comes from many different viewpoints, some radically different from my own. I have employed pseudonyms and omitted some identifying details, unless the interviewee gave explicit permission otherwise. In the interest of avoiding tokenism, I have also refrained from including supplementary information about an interviewee's age, race, sexual orientation, or gender identity unless she chose to specifically discuss these details within the context of the interview.

Much of this book is also inspired by my own years of personal experience with relationship experimentation, exploratory writing that I did for the blog at Multiamory.com, and the wealth of wisdom I've gained in my relationship coaching work. My clients also represent a vast diversity—pansexual, parents, swingers, singles, couples, triads, and more. Without getting too sentimental, every coaching session that I do is a blessing. The people who choose to work with me never fail to help me discover new insights for myself and my own relationships. Many of my clients have graciously agreed to have their stories shared within these pages.

Language Logistics

Though this book was written with the female experience in mind, I have tried to write inclusively rather than exclusively. You might be cis-gender or not. You might choose to present as femme or not. You might align yourself with any number of possible gender expressions in the vast and exquisite realm of identity. You might pick up this book with excitement because you personally identify as a "smart girl." You might be hesitant because you identify as a girl, you just don't have girl body parts. You may not identify as female, but the majority of your partners do, and you might be seeking to better understand their experience. Or you might be turning up your nose at the fact that I chose to use "girl" instead of "woman." Rest assured that this book makes no assumptions about your age, sexuality, gender identity, or relationship landscape.

When I make reference to "your partner," the term should be applied comprehensively to whichever interpersonal relationship the situation in context is most relevant to. "Your partner" may be a spouse, a boyfriend, a girlfriend, a one-night stand, a person you only see twice a year, or the person you raise children with. In the interest of pulling away from couple-centrism, "your partner" does not by default refer to one person you hold more important than anyone else, nor does it imply that is how your relationship life should be structured. "Your partner" may be one of several partners you currently enjoy.

Lastly, you will find a glossary in the back of the book to clarify any terminology that may be new to you. This glossary is far from exhaustive but will include most of the specialized vocabulary used here.

The Journey Begins

I am far from being the world's leading expert on polyamory or even human relationships. I'm still on that journey for myself. But my hope in this book is to empower you to become the expert on the subject of you, what you want, and what you love. By the time you finish this book, you may decide that your romantic journey will be polyamory, or it may be swinging, or it might even be consciously-chosen, long-term monogamy. But instead of looking outward to all those magazines, movies, and songs on the radio, you'll be on the journey of looking inward to create your own definitions of love and crafting your own totally unique vision of a healthy, happy love life. You may not be able to answer the question "What is love?" but you will be able to answer the more important questions—"What is love . . . *to me*? What do *I* do about it?"

Section I

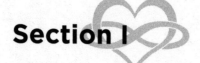

Polyamory 101

1 Polyamory: What It Is and What It Isn't

When I was a young adult and first started exploring romantic rela-tionships, I didn't put much thought into it. After all, a childhood of watching Disney movies and going to church every Sunday had taught me everything I needed to know about love and sex, or so I thought. You meet the boy, you fall deeply in love at first sight, you share true love's first kiss (with maybe some stray birds or little woodland animals happily observing), and you dutifully save your virginity until your wedding night, at which point you consummate your union and spend the remainder of your lives in wedded bliss plus kids. Easy.

Imagine my sheer confusion when, after being with my very first boyfriend for a few months, I found myself developing a crush on another boy.

Something is wrong! I'm in love with my boyfriend; how could I be developing feelings for someone else? The Disney movies hadn't covered this scenario. Once you fell in love with someone, that was it. Roll credits. You were so in love you didn't even want to look at anybody else. I thought that I was broken. I ended the relationship with my first boyfriend and cut off contact with the guy I was crushing on, convinced that I was very seriously messed up to fall in love with more than one person.

The next few years of my adult life were a string of serial monogamous relationships. I followed a repeating pattern of falling in love, settling into the relationship, and then unexpectedly finding myself infatuated with someone who was not my boyfriend. Cheating was not on the menu for me, so one of two things would happen: I would suffer extreme guilt over what I thought was a sign of flagging personal integrity and fall into a depression, or I would abandon my current relationship in order to pursue a connection with my new fancy. It's a pattern that is all too familiar to many people.

I was twenty-three when I finally grew sick of the cycle. Once again I had developed a crush on someone who wasn't my boyfriend. I didn't want to end the relationship. I didn't want to cheat. I didn't want to be miserable. So I did what was then unthinkable to me: I proposed opening the relationship.

Like many people, I thought that open relationships were only for commitment-phobes or sex addicts. But at this point of desperation, I started doing my research. Googling "open relationship" first exposed me to the word *polyamory*. I researched voraciously. It totally blew my mind that not only were there a lot of people doing this, they were doing it in a way that was viable, stable, and healthy. People were loving multiple people—and everyone was happy about it! So many assumptions that I had made about love, relationships, and even myself were turned upside down. It was confronting but exhilarating, and my stomach was both knotted up and full of butterflies when I finally pitched the idea to my boyfriend.

My first attempt went horribly.

I was a terrible communicator; he didn't *really* want to be in an open relationship, and after some sloppy attempts at being polyamorous, our relationship came to a close six months later. But *even* when it was miserable, *even* when I was making one mistake after another, I still felt like I had uncovered something huge. My brain continued to burn, unable to forget everything I had learned. There was no way I could go back to the relationships I had before.

Several years later, I've now met multiple people who have experienced the same phenomenon. Learning about polyamory (or ethical non-monogamy or relationship anarchy or any of the many other manifestations of alternative relationships) is for many a radical awakening into a whole new paradigm. Like seeing the Matrix. Often there is no going back, which for some means a future of only polyamorous relationships and for others means a very clear decision to consciously embrace monogamy.

This new awareness surrounding relationships and sex need not be conflated with an intellectual enlightenment or spiritual awakening (though frequently it is). Becoming conscious of your relationships means also becoming conscious of your needs, your fears, your desires, what you want for your future, and ultimately what makes you tick and makes you *you*. Call it seeing the Matrix, call it enlightenment, call it turning over a new leaf. But whatever you call it, know that the things you learn in this book and the things you learn about yourself along the way are impossible to unlearn.

Before getting too lofty, first things first—education. Back when I was first awakened to the possibility of consciously crafting my relationships, I had to hunt through Google search results to find online forums, book suggestions, and random personal blog posts on polyamory buried in some corner of the

Internet. Today, there is a wide variety of excellent informational resources on all different types of non-monogamy. This chapter will walk you through the fundamentals of polyamory in its myriad different forms, as well as address some common misconceptions that may arise about polyamory, women, and the nature of love itself.

What It Is

Ask any random person to define the word *love*, and you are guaranteed a unique and revealing answer. The same goes for the word *polyamory*. At its very simplest, it breaks down linguistically:

poly = many

amory = loves

This definition is simple, but even a description this reductive is controversial. (Mostly among linguaphiles, since the word commits the linguistic no-no of mixing Greek and Latin roots.)

But the devil is in the details. "Many loves" is broad and inclusive, and consequently polyamorous communities often debate what actually counts as having "many loves." As more people become aware of alternatives to monogamy, more questions are arising. If you're casually dating many partners but not planning on getting into any long-term relationships, does that count as polyamory? What about a couple who is emotionally monogamous, but sexually non-monogamous, such as swingers? If you had a threesome with your boyfriend once, but the two of you normally never have sex with anyone else, can you still label your relationship as monogamous? Is there a difference between being in an open relationship and self-identifying as polyamorous?

What's in a Name?

Labels and definitions can be a double-edged sword. No one wants to be hedged in by a narrow, oversimplified categorization, but it's also useful to have a go-to word that will quickly and easily identify yourself and your relationships. Alternative relationships are gaining visibility, which on the plus side means that people are now more likely to understand what you mean if you tell them, "I'm polyamorous." On the other hand, this also means people are more likely to have preconceived notions of what *polyamory* or *open relationship* might mean. These ideas could be shaped by the media, their church, or whatever gossip they heard from their coworker. I've spent many years telling people that I'm polyamorous, but even that requires a follow-up conversation where I specify what that means to me and what that looks like in my life. Even if you decide to commit to polyamory, you will always have to clarify what it means to you, even to other poly folk.

In the 1940s and '50s, Alfred Kinsey's research shook up conventional ideas about sexuality with the introduction of the Kinsey scale. Kinsey posited that human beings, rather than being categorized as strictly heterosexual or homosexual, fell along a scale of sexual preference.[1] Today, the spectrum between heterosexual and homosexual has been populated by numerous terms: bisexual, heteroflexible, pan- or omnisexual, bi-curious, sexually fluid—the list goes on and on. In much the same way, the simple definition of "many loves" has been the subject of much fine tuning and tweaking to become more specific and serve a wide variety of relationship structures. New terms are rapidly being coined to support multiple flavors of relationship format and identity.

A collection of specific terms and unique relationship structures and practices will be covered later in the book, but here I want to introduce the three most commonly used and generally understood labels—*non-monogamy, polyamory,* and *open relationship*—and clarify the definitions that will be used for them from here on.

non-monogamy—any relationship structure that is not based on sexual or romantic exclusivity

I use *non-monogamy* as a wide umbrella term that includes every variety of polyamory, swinging, couples who are "monogamish,"[2] nonexclusive Dom/sub dynamics, etc.—any relationship structure that is not defined by sexual exclusivity to a single partner. Some people prefer to specifically say *ethical* or *consensual* non-monogamy to philosophically distance themselves from what may be the most culturally familiar yet morally questionable form of non-monogamy: cheating. Any reference to non-monogamy in this book is inclusive of ethical, consensual, and honest relationship structures. It is frustrating that there has yet to be a thorough term for these relationships other than pointing out what they are *not*.

polyamory—engaging in multiple romantic relationships simultaneously with full knowledge and consent of all partners involved

This is the basic meaning that will be used throughout this book, but keep in mind that within polyamory there are many gradients, which will be discussed in more detail. These multiple relationships may be short-term or long-term, deeply intimate or more casual, sexual or nonsexual. Frequently, a polyamorist may be in multiple relationships that represent a vast variety of relationship depth, format, attachment, and life entwinement.

open relationship—a dyadic (two-person) relationship wherein each partner is free to pursue other partners sexually or romantically

Including a definition for _open relationship_ may seem repetitive. An open relationship is by definition non-monogamous and could also be polyamorous in nature. I include it here because I've found it to be the most accessible and frequently used term in Western culture. If someone has never heard of polyamory or ethical non-monogamy, chances are they are at least familiar with the concept of an open relationship. Often, couples who were previously in a monogamous, "closed" relationship will refer to their relationship as having _opened up_ rather than as being _polyamorous._

First Encounters

Most of us grow up learning that monogamy is the default for romantic relationships. It is modeled over and over again in most popular magazines, books, and movies, especially those that are marketed to young women and girls. For most people, our parents served as the most influential example of the potential effectiveness (or ineffectiveness) of marriage and lifetime monogamy. In a culture that primarily presents monogamy as the only viable option for happy relationships, it is difficult to organically encounter examples of alternatives without specifically searching for them.

I got curious about women who chose to break away from established cultural norms and seek something different. How did they come across the possibility of polyamory? What opened them up to ethical non-monogamy? The wide range of first access points is surprising—from witnessing Islamic polygamy to encountering poly community members in an online game! Even in monogamous cultures, alternatives can show up in unexpected places.

❝*I have a friend of mine who tried to court me while I was in the infancy of my current relationship (three years in or so). He also had a girlfriend, and I would get mad at him because he would flirt with me knowing full well he was taken. He then explained to me what polyamory was and how his family was of that nature. His mom had a boyfriend; his dad had a girlfriend. His parents would often travel to visit their other significant others. Actually, his dad's girlfriend lived with them after a while. It opened my eyes. It dawned on me that this is something that exists.* **❞**—Anna

❝*I spent some time as a young woman (12–15) living in Pakistan, and one of the features of Islam is the ability to have multiple wives, provided each of the women you're already married to agrees, and provided you can "keep" them equally. This is technically polygamy, but I remember at that age thinking that there wasn't so much wrong with that because, compared to Mormon polygamy for example, there was no belief that a woman could only seek God through her husband. The element of consent really attracted me as well—I guess at that point I had a very "live and let live" mentality on the subject, but I still practiced monogamy in my own relationships.* **❞**—Lila

❝*I first heard about polyamory when I was thirteen on an MTV show called* Undressed. *At the time, I was first recognizing my bisexuality (and first putting language to it) and knew that I couldn't be fully satisfied with a partner of only one gender. As such, my first girlfriend and I decided that we would open our relationship so that we could have male partners but would be each other's only female partners.* **❞**—Kat

❝ *The word caught in my head, and I couldn't wait to get home to Google the heck out of it and dredge up any information I could about the subject. It made so much sense to me; I always had trouble with monogamous relationships in high school, and I'd begin to have feelings for other people while being in a relationship. I was always forced to choose one or the other, because monogamy is the standard. It felt like a door had been opened to me, and I couldn't wait to talk about it with my boyfriend.* **❞**—Alina

❝*I had heard the term [polyamory] before several times but never really came into solid contact with meaning to the term until I was in a guild in* World of Warcraft *that had two poly couples that were also deeply involved in the BDSM scene. Through the two couples sort of raising me, as it were, in the BDSM and poly scene, I had grown to learn a lot about the benefits and drawbacks. I later came to accept that both were entirely for me.* **❞**—Julie

The starting points for each of these journeys are different, but the common element is a sense of realization—that it is possible to deviate from the norms set down for women and for their relationships. Women who make the choice to color outside the lines are courageous, considering that going beyond the bounds of normalcy is rarely the path of least resistance. Before examining the female experience of alternative relationships, it is important to observe the traditional context surrounding relationships and sex in which women are expected to operate.

Female Fairy Tales

There are a number of ingrained cultural beliefs about the inherent nature of women and how women should relate to love and sex. Both men and women are socialized based on templates for behavior that remain largely unquestioned. It is usually taken as a given that men are sexually enthusiastic, sometimes to an uncontrollable extent, and a large number of casual sex partners is appealing to the average guy. On the flip side, women are expected to be passive, coy, and to seek out sex only within an emotionally committed context. These gender-normative templates are established and reinforced by religion, advertising, mass media, and often our own families and peer groups.

Sigmund Freud first coined the term *Madonna-whore complex* to describe the phenomenon wherein men categorize women as either Madonnas (pure, wholesome, virginal, motherly) or whores (sexualized, slovenly, licentious). The paradox is that while the stereotypical man admires, respects, and loves Madonna women, he is hopelessly attracted to the whore, and desires her sexually despite holding little respect for her.[3] Today, Freud's theories have largely been disproved, abandoned, or categorically thrown out the window. However, the Madonna-whore complex can still be seen in the way that women are conditioned to approach relationships and sex.

It's expected that no woman wants to be the whore, at least not if she is seeking stable relationships. That means the only option is to be a Madonna. The problem is that the character of the Madonna is its own contradiction. How can a woman be a virgin and a mother at the same time? Immaculate conceptions just don't happen as frequently as they used to!

Since few sexually active women identify entirely as whores or entirely as Madonnas, there is now a landscape rife with several centuries' worth of conflicting advice. Never sleep with a man on the first date. But also don't be frigid and withhold sex for too long, or he might abandon you for someone else. Don't admit the number of sexual partners you've had. However, if you don't have sexual experience and know-how before getting into bed with him, he'll be turned off. Stay sexually attractive by working out, putting on the right makeup, doing your hair, and wearing flattering clothes, but don't appear too eager by actually pursuing someone. Let him send the first text, make the first move, and chase you to the ends of the earth in order to realize how worthy of love and attention you are. Wrapped up in all of this is, of course, the unattainably high standards for beauty and personal appearance supported by our culture at large.

There has been a growing movement, largely fueled by third-wave feminism, to fight back against these expectations in the name of female empowerment. Women, tired of decades of being sexualized, objectified, and trivialized, are speaking up, and content creators and advertisers are starting to listen. Solid female characters are being more frequently written into popular TV shows and movies. The past few decades have seen some advertisers breaking the mold and running "real beauty" campaigns or portraying women as strong, active, and capable (although keep in mind that advertisers are still primarily motivated by selling products rather than advancing female empowerment).

This movement is making its way into the realm of dating and relationships. In Western culture we are now long past the days of the man being expected to pay for every date or ask a woman's father for permission to court her. We can now witness the growing embrace of sex positivity as well as the controversial "hookup culture" that is characterized by its popularity among college-aged women. The new "empowered" message to young women is: focus on your own goals and fuck whomever you want, whenever you want, no strings attached (as long as you settle down eventually).

Hookup culture, sex positivity, and the feminist reclamation of casual sex will be discussed more in chapter 6, but I want to make it clear that this book is not encouraging any woman to cast off a history of sexual oppression by throwing all discretion to the wind. "Playing like the boys do" by appropriating cavalier and typically "macho" attitudes toward sex does not equal advancement toward women's sexual liberation.

In the middle ground between the traditional romantic passivity and the aggressively modern hookup culture are the women who choose polyamory. Not conforming to one-size-fits-all monogamy but also not hopping into a sexual free-for-all, these women are in a middle ground that is frequently misunderstood, misrepresented, and straight-up baffling to traditional culture at large. In a world where you're either single or taken, a faithful partner or a rotten cheater, it is difficult for non-monogamous women to find acknowledgment, tolerance, and understanding.

In-group vs. Out-group

The unfortunate reality is that society is rarely understanding toward those who don't fit neatly into boxes. This is simply the way the human brain is built—we process our environment by simplifying it. We simplify the environment by categorizing it. This means dividing people into social groups. In order to differentiate social groups even further, we mentally exaggerate the positive qualities of our in-group (the group we belong to) and the negative qualities of the out-group (those weirdos over there).[4] This psychology can fall on a wide spectrum—everything from staunch loyalty to your favorite football team (*We're number 1!!*) to genocide (*The Jews must be exterminated*).[5]

Polyamory defies the rules of standard relationships, but has not yet become widely known or accepted, leaving poly and non-monogamous folks open to all kinds of interpretations. Some misinterpretations can be offensive, some are downright comical, and many highlight exactly what an alternative relationship *isn't*. Some people perceive the very existence of polyamory to be a threat to their own practice of monogamy and may make some nasty comparisons, all in the name of distinguishing the in-group from the out-group.

What It Isn't

My partners and polyamorous friends often lament the hazards of giving "The Talk"—the speech explaining polyamory and non-monogamy to those new to it. It is often a long-winded, conversation-dominating monologue that invariably ends in a rigorous question-and-answer session that fascinates some, disgusts others, and annoys the hell out of everyone else around who already knows what polyamory is. For years I've threatened to put together a PowerPoint presentation and hand it out on flash drives, but I decided to write this book instead.

Let's examine some of the most common misconceptions that come up in The Talk. If you are reading this book, chances are you already have a little bit of familiarity with polyamory, but some of these thoughts may be running through your head as you learn more about it. See if any of these sound familiar—either from that little voice inside or from other people.

That's the weird thing Mormons do, right?

Say the word *polyamory* and you'll find it how easy it is for people to mentally leap to *polygamy*. Due to the right combination of mystery and scandal, the Mormon church has a nearly two-hundred-year history of being associated with polygamy as a spiritual practice. In reality, the Church of Jesus Christ of Latter Day Saints condemned plural marriage in an official statement over 100 years ago, but certain fundamentalist sects still practice it.[6] The typical pop culture image of a Mormon polygamist evokes a man (usually older and heavily bearded) surrounded by multiple devout wives, some of whom may be extremely young. The controversial history of the Mormon church and its influence on American attitudes toward multi-partner relationships will be explained further in chapter 2.

However, it comes down to semantics. This practice is actually better described by the term *polygyny*—having multiple female partners. In fundamentalist Mormonism, women are strictly forbidden from pursuing other male partners.[7] *Polygamy* refers to being married to multiple spouses, who could be of either gender. While concurrent marriage is currently outlawed in many countries, the legalization of secular polygamy is becoming a talking point within non-monogamous communities (see chapter 11).

The choice to have polyamorous relationships rarely has to do directly with one's spirituality or religious expression. Healthy relationships also do not typically restrict one or multiple partners to monogamy while the other gets to have as many non-monogamous relationships as he or she likes. (Some monogamous people do willingly choose to partner with a polyamorous person, a format discussed in depth in chapter 8.) Shows like *Big Love* and *Sister Wives* have opened up many Americans to the possible benefits of having multiple partners, but unfortunately these relationships are only presented in this specifically religious and one-sided package.

Is this a kinky sexual thing?

Sex is a charged topic. In Western culture we have a long history of being both sexually repressed and sexually obsessed. Our modern-day attitudes toward sex are a mixed bag of scandal, enticement, temptation, and shame. The sexual aspect of nontraditional relationships without a doubt draws the most questions and also causes the most offended reactions.

Under the broad umbrella of *non-monogamy*, breaking out of the exclusive two-person-relationship model is often driven by sex. For example, a couple may regularly go to sex parties or swingers' parties, which may be an agreed-upon safe space to sexually explore with other people. Outside of these specific spaces and events, however, the couple may practice emotional and sexual monogamy. Because multiple partners are only a part of the couple's sexual play, they will likely choose not to disclose this facet of their private lives to family and friends. Another example would be the "100-mile rule" that some couples establish, where casual hook-ups and sexual flings are allowed, but only when one or both partners are out of town or traveling separately from each other.

It is a different story with polyamorous relationships. Because the emphasis is on building and nurturing romantic relationships, there is much more than sexual exploration at play. The sexual side of polyamorous relationships represents only one part of the whole, and this part can look many different ways. Three people who are in a triad relationship may sexually engage with each other on an individual basis or all together in a threesome. Alternately, a person may have multiple partners and multiple sexual dynamics within each of those individual relationships, but those partners do not also have sex with each other.

The sex in any given polyamorous relationship may be defined by leather-bondage, acrobatic, off-the-wall kinkiness, or by gentle, cuddly, missionary-style vanilla. The full spectrum is possible, just as it is with the average monogamous relationship. The important takeaway here is that polyamory is not just a sexual fetish, nor is it limited to the realm of sexual exploration. A much more in-depth exploration of sexuality in poly relationships can be found in chapter 6.

Misconceptions versus Judgments

Clearing up misconceptions about your lifestyle or chosen type of relationship generally leads to better understanding overall. Once you've painted a clear picture of your love life, many people will be curious or politely neutral. Unfortunately, some people will react with harsh judgments, such as:

You're being a slut.
What you're doing is immoral.
This is sinful.
You're sick.

Judgments like these are not as easy to neutralize as misconceptions. Misconceptions arise from a lack of awareness and information, but judgments come from an individual's value system, definitions of right and wrong, and perception of how the world is supposed to work. Chapter 9 will cover negative or judgmental reactions from others and how to handle them with grace and smarts.

So you're just playing the field for now?

The standard rituals of dating and courtship in the twenty-first century have developed into a reliable pattern. One is either *single*—not in a committed monogamous relationship—or *taken*—in a committed monogamous relationship. Being single means having the freedom to date around, play the field, see just how many different types of fish in the sea there are. Ironically, the ultimate goal of dating is to eventually stop dating . . . but only after you've found Mr. Right.

Dating around is one of the few arenas where non-monogamy is culturally accepted, though with chagrin. After all, you're exploring your options! In this period it's considered good taste to not be explicitly honest about the number of other people that you're dating or to give any details as to the nature of those developing relationships. Depending on how many dating partners you have and how long you choose to draw this out, it can turn into quite a juggling game—lying to a partner by saying that you're out "with friends" when you're actually out on a date, or scrambling to tidy up your place so that the next person coming over won't see any evidence of last night's roll in the hay with someone else. Once the "right" person comes along, all other dating pursuits must be nipped in the bud in order to focus on developing an exclusive relationship. For this reason, dating relationships have to be kept at arm's length, without much intimacy or emotional bonding. The go-to phrase? *I want to keep things casual. I don't want to be committed right now.*

This juggling game works for some, but it drives me crazy.

By contrast, effective polyamorous and non-monogamous relationships are distinguished by total honesty with all of your partners about the other people that you're dating, having sex with, or in a relationship with. The level of detail and type of information shared is determined by the individuals within each particular relationship, but no one is hiding certain partners or interactions from other partners.

These relationships are also different from casual dating in that the goal is not to find The One to settle down with. Falling in love with someone new does not mean abandoning all other relationships. And rarely is polyamory a transitory phase while in between "real" relationships.

Isn't that just cheating?

Within the confines of a monogamous relationship, any non-monogamous behavior can be construed as cheating. Infidelity is traditionally defined as engaging in sexual contact with someone who is not your romantic partner, but some may add flirting, growing too emotionally close with someone outside of the relationship, or even checking out other people to the list. On the surface, a relationship in which sex and intimacy is shared with more than one person can bear a striking resemblance to cheating.

However, it is important to think outside the box when getting to the heart of what cheating actually is. In 2007, Oscar award-winning actress Mo'Nique publicly revealed her open marriage. In the years following, media outlets jumped all over this news, and headlines claimed that she gives her husband "a free pass to cheat." In 2015, Mo'Nique clarified many details about her relationship and addressed the accusations of free-for-all cheating. "We don't give each other passes to cheat, because when you cheat, you lie, when you lie, you steal."[8,9] Cheating is non-monogamy, but it is also nonconsensual.

Cheating incorporates an element of cloak-and-dagger beyond just having sex with multiple people. When you cheat, you are taking actions that go against the fundamental agreements of your relationship, and usually this is followed by some form of dishonesty in order to cover it up. This means that infidelity can look different depending on the agreements of each different relationship. If you and your partner have agreed to be sexually and emotionally exclusive to each other, then falling in love or having sex with someone else is cheating. If you and your partner have agreed to be non-monogamous but always communicate honestly with each other about your individual dating lives, then lying or omitting information about starting a new relationship could be cheating.

Regardless of the type of relationship, it is important to clearly communicate what you consider to be infidelity. Don't assume that you already know what would upset your partner or that your partner already knows what would upset you! I've witnessed monogamous relationships go for years before having this conversation, which usually occurs after one partner violates an unknown, unspoken rule. Talk about this early and often!

Once you find the right person, you'll stop wanting to sleep around with other people.

Many people believe that if you're *really* in love, you'll lose all desire or interest in anyone other than the object of your affections. When you fall in love with someone and you're experiencing that intense chemical rush known as *new relationship energy*, it can be easy to forget about everything else, including friends, family, hobbies, and even obligations to school or work! For a while, it really does feel the way they show it in the movies.

However, this does not mean that you are incapable of being attracted to or feeling affection for other people. You don't stop feeling love for your brother or lose your desire to hang out with your best friend when you start falling in love with someone else, yet for some reason we expect that any romantic or sexual feelings for anyone else will be instantly canceled out by our existing romantic or sexual feelings.

This expectation has caused distress for many people. The truth is, whether you are in the exciting beginning stages of a new relationship or if you are happily and solidly bonded to someone after several years, it is still quite possible *and totally normal* to feel attraction to others. Human beings are built for a lifetime of reproduction—it just makes sense that we would maintain our ability to be turned on by as many other people as possible. As the authors of the popular "Bible" of polyamory, *The Ethical Slut*, say: a wedding ring around the finger does not cause a nerve block to the genitals.[10]

So what does this mean for you? If you're monogamous, don't let attraction to another person cause you to doubt the love and desire you have for your current partner, and don't let your partner's attraction to other people be a source of anxiety or threat. If you're polyamorous, rejoice in being able to talk your partners about who you're attracted to and get excited about their new squeeze as well!

There's only one person out there who is your soul mate. Why waste your time with someone who is not The One?

Romantic love has had a long evolution before becoming what it is to us today. The search for "The One" or your "soul mate" is popular and highly romanticized. The idea is that there is one person out there who is meant for you. When you meet this person, the stars will align, you will be completed, and according to some, the relationship will not be difficult or require any work because of how perfectly and divinely matched you are. This concept was first seen in Plato's *Symposium*.

In Plato's philosophical allegory, the character of Aristophanes delivers a speech describing the origins of romantic love. He claims that in the beginning of time, human beings had two sets of body parts—two heads, two mouths, four legs, double sets of genitalia, etc. When the gods grew uneasy about the growing power of these beings, they decided to split them each in half and scatter them to the winds. Aristophanes concludes that since that time, man is "always looking for his other half."[11]

There is no denying that the story is romantic. How could you not be ecstatic to meet another person who undeniably connects with you, understands you, and loves you in a way that transcends the limitations of time and space? Some of us have experienced a connection like this, and some have yet to. When you do build a relationship based on this kind of connection, it is game-changing, disruptive, and unforgettable.

I'm of the opinion that these connections are not limited to once in a lifetime. Some are blessed by The One, and others are blessed by The Many. In my life, some connections have opened my eyes to how deep and earth-shattering intimacy can be, and others have challenged me and woken me up to my faults and my strengths. Having multiple partners does not mean you are sacrificing the dream of finding a soul mate or that you don't believe in true love. Tikva Wolf writes in her poly and genderqueer comic *Kimchi Cuddles*, "I just didn't stop looking for the other [soul mates] after I found the first one!"[12]

And who's to say that before the gods split us apart, there weren't some of us wandering around with three or four sets of body parts? (More disturbing to visualize, but just as romantic.)

That's not a real relationship, and that's not real love.

The definition of "love" is already quite sticky, much less defining what counts as "real" love or a "real" relationship. Some say a relationship is only real if it leads to marriage and kids. Others say a relationship is real after he or she has met your parents. And still others maintain that a real relationship means you never fight with each other.

Many popular women's publications have published advice on how to tell if you're in a "for-real" relationship. Commonly mentioned indicators include making plans for the future with your partner, spending the holidays together, and losing all desire or interest for anyone else.[13,14] Ultimately, these publications uphold the steadfast belief that long-term monogamous relationships are the only type of relationship worthy of pursuit and effort. Anything outside of that is not a "real" relationship.

Most of us are raised to believe that love is infinite, but not when it comes to romance. A mother can love multiple children, a person can love multiple friends, but you can't truly love more than one romantic partner. There's this belief that romantic love is a limited resource, and if you give it to multiple people, you must be taking it away from someone else.

Just like love for your family or love for your friends, romantic love is infinite. It can be abundantly given to as many people as you want without losing power or intensity. What *is* finite is time and money. In a competitive and capitalist culture, it's possible that we've started to misconstrue time and money as symbols of love.

Without getting too metaphysical, it's important to know that love is an illogical force that operates outside of the seemingly logical limits of time, space, and money. The father who only has a poverty-line income to provide for his kids doesn't love them less because his money is limited. The soldier who has been on deployment doesn't love her husband any less because she has only seen him once in the past year. You can lie in bed next to the same person every night for twenty years and not feel an iota of love or compassion for them. Do not think that all love needs physical proximity, disposable income, or 100 percent of your time in order to be real.

When you start looking at love in this way, you begin to realize that you have access to an extremely powerful force of good, a limitless and abundant resource, a transcendent instrument that can nurture, heal, and light up sparks in yourself and anyone else you meet. You're like a superhero, rockstar, and Jedi Master all rolled up in one! Who wouldn't want to bring that kind of power to every relationship?

You can't actually be happy this way.

It should be obvious that the only person who knows if you are happy or not is *you*. Don't let anybody—your partner, your parents, your therapist, your boss, *anybody*—tell you that you are unhappy when you are actually happy. There are many paths to happiness, peace, and contentment, and they all look different. If your actions are safe, healthy, positive, and not causing harm, you get the privilege of creating and owning your path to happiness.

Lesbian author Jeannette Winterson ironically poses the question, "Why be happy when you could be normal?"[15] Ultimately it is your decision how much "normal" you need to sacrifice in order to be happy. I'm firmly of the belief that giving up normalcy in exchange for fulfillment and joy is always worth it.

At the end of the day, no one can argue with your happiness. So go find it and don't let anyone tell you it should be otherwise!

You Can't Make This Stuff Up

These misconceptions aren't as common, but they are too ridiculous not to mention.

Does that mean you're a cult leader?

That's a brilliant idea! You keep every girl jealous of each other, so they'll all try extra hard to be prettier and better in bed!

You must have orgies and threesomes all the time.

All polyamorous people are bisexual, and all bisexual men are secretly gay. Therefore, a polyamorous man dating multiple women must be gay.

Your soul mate's spirit must have been destroyed in another life.

Chapter 1 Homework

Exercise #1

Think about your earliest memories, probably from around the time you were three or four. What were your earliest thoughts about romantic love? What about relationships? Sex? Were these things positive or negative? Did you learn about them from your parents, your friends, by watching a movie?

Exercise #2

Think about all the stereotypes, positive and negative, that you know about women. It will probably be easy to come up with several, but here are a few common ones to get you started:

- *Women don't enjoy sex as much as men.*
- *Women just want to get married and settle down.*
- *Women only date jerks.*
- *Women are better at negotiating and making compromises.*

For each stereotype, make two lists: women you know (personally or not) who live up to these stereotypes and women who defy them. How many of these stereotypes do you see in yourself? How many do you see yourself defying?

Exercise #3

Let's reexamine Jeanette Winterson's quote.

Why be happy when you could be normal?

In what ways are you or your life not "normal" by outside standards? Is there anything that you wish you could do or a way you wish you could be that you avoid pursuing because it isn't "normal"?

2 From Tribal Living to Sacred Cuddling Parties: The Unwritten History of Polyamory

In 1986, anthropologists unearthed a prehistoric grave near Dolni Vestonice in the Czech Republic. The area was already renowned for containing many Paleolithic artifacts and remains, but this 25,000-year-old burial site was particularly unique. It contained the skeletons of three individuals, two men and one woman, lying side by side. Their bodies seem to have been buried with intention and ritual. The man to the right of the woman shows evidence of a traumatic skull injury and was buried facedown with his head turning away, but his left arm is linked with the woman's right. The man on the woman's left is reaching for her pelvis with both hands, and his hip has been impaled by a wooden stake or spear. Each of their heads and the pelvis of the woman are decorated with red ochre.[1] Evidently, some kind of story is being told in the way these ancient humans were laid to rest, but what could it be?

In his book *Anatomy of Desire*, an examination of human psychology surrounding sex and marriage, author Simon Andreae cites the burial as the earliest evidence of ritualistic punishment for infidelity. Andreae paints a narrative of the man on the right being the cuckolded husband of the woman, looking away from her in shame. The man on the left is the interloper, possibly executed along with the adulteress in the middle. Andreae argues that this is clear evidence that human beings always have and always will seek to protect and maintain monogamy as the status quo.[2]

But Andreae's story is only one of dozens of interpretations. Some anthropologists postulate that the woman in the center may have died during childbirth (hence the decoration on her pelvis). The two men flanking her are her husband and a midwife or shaman, who were put to death for failing to save the woman's life. Still other scientists have found evidence to suggest that the three individuals may actually be siblings, and there are even some theories that the skeleton in the middle may not be female after all but may have belonged to an intersex individual. It's been a long time since my Anthropology 101 class, but I could throw in my own hypothesis that the burial depicts a polyamorous triad relationship that ended tragically in some kind of inter-tribal conflict.

The point is that when we look to the past, searching early human history for clues as to the origins of our modern-day behaviors, there's a lot of ambiguity. We have scraps of evidence—bone fragments, pottery shards, cave paintings—and only analysis and imagination to fill in the missing puzzle pieces. Analysis and imagination can take us far in solving the mysteries of the past, but they are dangerously susceptible to *confirmation bias*—interpreting ambiguous data in a way that supports an existing belief, hypothesis, or expectation.[3]

Is the mysterious triple burial of Dolni Vestonice empirical proof that human beings have always prioritized monogamy? Or does it undoubtedly confirm that early tribes of humans practiced polyamory? There's no way to know for sure either way. The most important thing to remember is that your current feelings toward sexuality, relationships, and fidelity can color your interpretations of the past. *Evolutionary psychology*—examining the evolutionary origins of our modern-day psychology—is particularly vulnerable to this.

For years, evolutionary psychology has been used to promote the notion that long-term monogamy and marriage are natural and biologically hard-wired into us, but newer research is uncovering that this may not be the case. However, proponents from both sides of the argument can be subject to confirmation bias, regardless of how objective they may claim to be. The best way to avoid being swayed by bias is to apply critical thinking. Check the source of the information, find other opinions and interpretations, read up on the subject matter, and don't take anyone's theoretical interpretations as solid fact. (Even mine.)

In this chapter, we'll look at the origins and colorful history of both monogamy and polyamory, making a through-line from the behavior of early human tribes to the modern-day polyamory community. You'll find that non-monogamy is far from being a new fad, but it couldn't have become what it is today without the right domino pieces of human adaptation, feminist movements, and sexual revolutions falling at just the right time. History nerds, it's time to buckle your seatbelts.

Pervasive Patriarchy?

In *Sex at Dawn: The Prehistoric Origins of Modern Sexuality*, authors Christopher Ryan and Cacilda Jetha cite an excellent example of confirmation bias at play. The Minangkabau tribe of Indonesia is primarily matriarchal, with women controlling inheritance of land, acting as head of the family line, and holding equal if not greater weight than the men do when making important decisions for the community. But scientists have repeatedly reported that the Minangkabau are patriarchal. The main evidence? The scientists, many of whom had already hypothesized that patriarchy was inevitable in all societies, observed that men were usually served food first and concluded that the Minangkabau must be patriarchal.

Adam and Eve

In my church-going days, the format for romantic relationships was cut and dried. In the beginning, God created man. Upon seeing that man was extremely unentertaining on his own, God created woman to spice things up. Man and woman had no choice but to find each other agreeable, and the model for human pair bonding was born. (Some artistic license taken in the re-telling.)

This model was reinforced by multiple examples in the Bible, albeit with some glossing over of the wife- and concubine-collecting habits of Abraham, Jacob, David, and other holy celebrities. Christian doctrine has greatly shaped the moral landscape of Western culture, but many other cultures and religions claim that human beings have been heterosexually monogamous from the dawn of time.

But let's shake off religious beliefs and mythic origin stories. Diving into the world of evolutionary psychology means dropping the stories handed to us by our culture and examining the behavior of our biological relatives and ancestors. This whole long-term romantic monogamy thing . . . who started it? For that answer, we need to look back in time before humans even became humans.

The Wayback Machine

Nonhuman primates don't exactly do the whole song and dance of first dates and marriage proposals (as far as we can tell). How is it that out of a world of mostly non-monogamous creatures, human beings came to seek monogamy and formalized relationships? Let's take a look at our closest primate relatives: chimpanzees and bonobos. We share 99 percent of our DNA with these two species. Chimpanzees are known to be aggressive and competitive, practicing infanticide and warmongering. On the other hand, bonobos are typically painted as being peaceful, relaxed, and horny enough to get it on with every other bonobo in the social group in every possible hetero- or homosexual configuration.[4,5]

There's been a long-standing debate among scientists as to which ape lent us the most behavioral traits. Human beings have a demonstrable history of violent behavior, but we also tend to seek peace and harmony in social groups. Like chimpanzees, we have a competitive streak—for jobs, mates, resources— and yet we are also interested in sex. So much so that we happily mate outside of the window of female fertility and for recreational reasons other than producing offspring, much like bonobos. Whether or not sexual partners are competed for or freely shared with everyone else, it's important to note that neither of these primates practice anything resembling lifelong monogamy, and it is unlikely that our early human ancestors did either.

Between observing primates and the behaviors witnessed in the few remaining hunter-gatherer communities on the planet, we can infer that it is likely that early humans lived in small nomadic tribes. These groups might occasionally stay in one spot for a particular season, and maybe even cultivate land on a small scale, but primarily they were mobile. Because these tribes were constantly on the move, there wasn't a lot of personal property to be found. Food that was hunted or gathered would be eaten immediately and generally shared with everyone else in the group. A person who hoarded food probably would have been shamed and ostracized.[6] Anthropologists now refer to this as *fierce egalitarianism*—sharing with the group is compulsory.[7] It was probably not as utopian and stress-free as you might be imagining, but cooperation and sharing was ultimately more beneficial for our ancestors than fierce competition.

Scientists argue that monogamous pair bonding allowed human females to secure and guard a mate who was good at providing food and who could take care of her offspring. Human babies are extremely vulnerable and weak, compared to the babies of other mammals, and having another pair of hands to help is necessary. The male would know that his partner's children were his, mitigating the risk that he'd be expending effort to help someone else pass on their genes. However, this makes the assumption that finding an exclusive male mate would be the female's *only* chance at surviving and raising her children successfully.

When you're in a culture where your grandparents, your aunts and uncles, your best friends, your cousins, and everyone else in your social network is contributing to the mutual care of you and everyone else, landing that one awesome male for a mate is not as high-stakes. Most hunter-gatherer societies have an equal division of labor, meaning that men and women have relatively equal power when it comes to feeding and taking care of the tribe.[8] You're able to provide for yourself, and you've already got everyone else watching your back as far as food and childcare goes. Why stress about bagging a husband when you've already got a safety net?

America's Polyamorous Roots

When Christian missionaries and colonialists first encountered Native American tribal cultures, there was inevitably a clash of values. Though every tribe had a wide variety of differing traditions and practices, native attitudes toward spirituality, land use, and particularly sex and marriage were often a source of great shock to the Europeans who witnessed them. Some examples of traditional Native American relationship practices that look very nontraditional to us today:

- Men of the Lakota Sioux would sometimes choose to create a deep, committed bond with another man, known as *kola*. The two *kolapi* swore to care for each other for life, particularly in battle. Both men freely shared their wives with each other, and sometimes *kolapi* would marry sisters to reduce the chances of any ill will between their wives.[9]
- The Huron embraced having multiple partners and discouraged any public displays of jealousy. There were monogamous "marriages," but these tended to be short and sweet—it was not uncommon to have had twelve to fifteen spouses in one's lifetime. If an unmarried girl got pregnant, she simply picked whomever she liked best out of all of her lovers to be named the "official" father of the child.[10]

- Among the Pawnee people, both polygyny (a man having multiple female partners) and polyandry (a woman having multiple male partners) were common. Brothers sometimes shared a single wife, and sisters would share a husband.[11] When a Pawnee boy reached puberty, he would go to live with his older brother or uncle, whose wife would sexually initiate him into adulthood. He would stay on as a "junior husband" in the years leading up to his own marriage.[12]

More Farms, Less Free Love

If the average Paleolithic woman didn't really *need* a husband to survive, there had to be other factors that kick-started the establishment of monogamy and marriage. The lifestyle of the hunter-gatherer began shifting drastically around 10,000 BCE, a time that anthropologists refer to as the *agricultural revolution*. The era saw the invention of the wheel, writing, and numbers, but it was with the pivotal invention of the plow that human beings were able to farm on a scale that was previously impossible. Food production increased, populations exploded, and civilization was born.[13]

It is around this time that the concept of private property—so commonplace to us today—first arose and became a defining feature of human culture. With the ability to grow large amounts of food without needing help from everyone else, hoarding food and taking ownership of land became necessary to ensure survival. Humans went from living within the environment to owning it, from having a mobile existence of few possessions to a sedentary life of houses, villages, farms, and granaries. As the agrarian man began controlling and collecting more and more resources, it became important to be sure that his land and resources would be inherited by offspring that were guaranteed to be his. Since there was no DNA testing, the only way to be sure of paternity was to require monogamy, at least from women.[14]

Women, once relatively autonomous and equally valued contributors, joined the ranks of property to be owned. Cuckoldry was prevented by establishing the ideal feminine sexuality to be chaste and virtuous, simultaneously virginal and procreative. Marriage began not as a declaration of love nor a dedication of one's loyalty, but as a business contract—exchanging food, shelter, and care for a woman's ability to produce farmworkers and heirs. Owning multiple wives became a status symbol. Instead of a large cooperative tribe, humans started living in communities of extended nuclear families.[15]

As populations continued to grow from a surplus of food, these communities banded together and cities formed, bringing the development of the class system and massively organized religion. The establishment of the Church and its subsequent influence on Western thought and morality is a topic too massive to address here, but suffice to say women and women's sexuality have never exactly been celebrated by long-standing Abrahamic religions (Christianity, Judaism, and Islam). These religions emphasized the inherently unclean nature of human beings and sexuality became conflated with wanton sinfulness. By the time the Industrial Revolution was underway, even polygyny was largely frowned upon, and socially imposed monogamy became the standard. These values slowly spread to the rest of the world with the globalizing forces of colonization, trade, and missionary work.[16]

Today, our definition of a "normal" relationship is the result of thousands of years of cultural development and socialization favoring monogamy, heterosexuality, and sex-negative principles. The Norman Rockwell portrait of the happy nuclear family upheld by the strong foundation of monogamous marriage may seem ubiquitous, but it has come at the cost of centuries of controlling, manipulating, and limiting human sexuality.

So What?

So monogamy may not be natural for human beings; so what? We benefit from indoor plumbing, air conditioning, birth control, antibiotics, organized government, the concept of human rights, and a thousand other "unnatural" inventions and social constructs on a daily basis. Just because monogamy isn't natural, does that make it bad?

Of course monogamy is not inherently bad. Monogamy and sexual preference in general have unfortunately been wrapped up in the moral code of long-standing religious and political institutions that have historically sought to control and limit human behavior through guilt, threats, and sometimes even violence. Because of this, relationship structure and sexuality have become psychologically entangled with our sense of virtue and ethics. For so much of our recorded history, human beings have been taught that the only "good" kind of sex is heterosexual, procreative, vanilla, and within the context of a long-term monogamous relationship. Any sex that is only for pleasure, or shared between people of the same sex, or experienced outside of a monogamous marriage, has been labeled as categorically "bad."

Monogamy is just one relationship structure out of many possible choices, but for a long time it has been foisted on us as the only choice. Those seeking otherwise have been ostracized, punished, shamed, and seen as deviant. But although monogamy is steadfastly embedded in our social code, there have still been a number of non-monogamous thinkers and communities that have sprung up over the past centuries.

Fans of Fourier

The Industrial Revolution changed the lives and landscape of much of the Western world, introducing major advances in transportation, the nine-to-five workday, and hitherto unseen amounts of air pollution. In the early 1800s, French philosopher Charles Fourier began writing and publishing his radical views in rebellion against the industrialization of society. Fourier called for the creation of a utopian society that would abandon the nuclear family structure and abolish anything that repressed human desires, including sexuality. His ideals held that the only forbidden sexual acts were those that involved pain or force, but everything outside of that was perfectly acceptable, including homosexuality, fetishism, and non-monogamy. Fourier staunchly supported the liberation of women and may have been the first to coin the term *feminism*.[17] He even went so far as to predict that in the ideal future, each woman would have four lovers or husbands simultaneously. Then again, he also predicted that eventually six moons would orbit the earth, so I'm not holding my breath.[18]

Fourier's writings were simultaneously revolutionary, eccentric, and a little bit crazy. However, his beliefs, so diametrically opposed to the ideals put in place by the religious and social landscape of his day, were paramount in laying the foundations for modern-day feminism and the sexual revolution. Many self-proclaimed "Fourierists" attempted to create utopian intentional communities in America during the mid-1800s, with varying degrees of success.[19]

Mormon Non-monogamy

The Fourierist movement of the mid-1800s also saw the rise of Joseph Smith and the creation of the Mormon religion. The Mormons also engaged in non-monogamous relationships, but only in the format of one man being allowed to have many wives, as is made very clear in their Doctrine and Covenants:

"61 . . . *If any man espouse a virgin, and desire to espouse another, and the first give her consent, and if he espouse the second, and they are virgins, and have vowed to no other man, then is he justified; he cannot commit adultery for they are given unto him; for he cannot commit adultery with that that belongeth unto him and to no one else.*

62 And if he have ten virgins given unto him by this law, he cannot commit adultery, for they belong to him, and they are given unto him; therefore is he justified.

*63 But if one or either of the ten virgins, after she is espoused, shall be with another man, she has committed adultery, and shall be destroyed . . .***"**[20]

Mormons do not officially approve of plural marriage and the destruction of virgins today, but some fundamentalist groups still maintain the practice. Popular reality shows like *Sister Wives* have showcased the intimate details of polygynous marriage, educating many people about both the benefits and pitfalls of this type of relationship. This book does not condone one-sided, single-gender polyamory; however, these examples in popular media have helped to frame multi-partner relationships as being viable, if also dramatic and difficult.

Oneida: Sex and Silverware

The most notable and arguably most successful Fourierist venture was the Oneida Community. Founder and leader John Humphrey Noyes, citing Jesus's words that there would be no marriage in heaven, created the concept of *complex marriage*. Noyes claimed that all men and women on earth were already married to each other and could therefore freely enjoy a variety of romantic and sexual partners.

In 1848 Noyes established the Oneida Community—an intentional community of about 300 members who shared property, raised children communally, and were permitted to engage in multiple romantic and sexual partnerships.[21] Men were strongly encouraged to practice *male continence*, known to us today as "the pull-out method," in order to prevent unwanted pregnancies. Women were allowed to dress and style themselves in more masculine ways, make important decisions regarding community policy, and to pursue work in whatever field most attracted them. The community members created a wide variety of business ventures for income, their most successful being the production of silverware.[22]

The Oneida Community lasted a little over thirty years—significantly longer than most other Fourierist societies of the time, which historically dissolved after four or five years. The community's final dissolution came at the hand of many factors. Complex marriage was, in itself, a scandalous concept and became even more so as more information about the community leaked to the outside world. Noyes himself was the primary overseer of matchmaking and granting permission to those who wished to conceive. Rumor spread of Noyes encouraging older and more "devout" men and women of the community to begin sexual relationships with significantly younger teenaged members. There was strong debate within the community over when, how, and if this should even be practiced, and a political struggle broke out over who would be the next to step into positions of leadership and make these decisions after Noyes had stepped down. Outside clergymen gathered to protest the community, and a warrant was issued for Noyes's arrest, causing him to flee to Canada. He urged his followers to abandon the practice of complex marriage, and the Oneida Community came to an end.[23] The only remnant left is the Oneida Ltd. silverware company, still going strong today. Unsurprisingly, there isn't much mention of complex marriage on their website.[24]

Personal accounts from those who lived in the community vary from triumphant stories of sexual awaking and liberation[25] to complaints over the lack of personal autonomy in relationship choice and the pain of mothers being separated from their children.[26] In the end, even though the community was liberal for its time, it was Noyes's dogmatic control over his followers' sexual and romantic choices—even going so far as to forbid monogamy—that led to the demise of his utopia. The Oneida Community acted as a double-edged sword: it demonstrated that the radical notions of women in positions of power and nonexclusive relationships were feasible, but ultimately failed by attempting to impose harsh control over the behavior of its members.

The Bloomsbury Group

Though Noyes's female-empowered and sexually liberated community met its demise, it was not long before the women's suffrage movement took the stage.

The turn of the century also saw the introduction of condoms and other pro-phylactics to prevent unwanted pregnancy, which caused an uproar in religious institutions. Women began to relinquish tight corsets and neck-to-ankle gowns for the loose-cut and temptingly short frocks that became ubiquitous among flappers.[27] The stifling conventions of the Victorian era were abandoned by many modernist intellectuals of the time, particularly by the famous Blooms-bury Group—a group of London-based writers and artists including author Virginia Woolf and her sister, painter Vanessa Bell, poet T. S. Eliot, and acclaimed economist Maynard Keynes (he's the guy to thank for giving us Keynesian economics).[28]

The Bloomsbury Group were not an intentional community per se, but they were once wryly described as "living in squares, painting in circles, and loving in triangles." The observation is apt, as the members of the Blooms-bury Group were entwined in a tight web of polyamorous relationships that explored the full spectrum of sexuality and gender identity. Virginia Woolf is well-known for frequently engaging in relationships with women outside of her marriage.[29] Her sister Vanessa Bell married the art critic Clive Bell, but both openly carried on multiple relationships outside of their marriage. Vanessa had children both with her husband Clive and her lover Duncan Grant, a bisex-ual painter who was also in romantic relationships with other Bloomsbury members Maynard Keynes and historian Lytton Strachey.[30] Strachey himself was living in an open triad relationship with painter Dora Carrington and her husband Ralph Partridge.[31]

Keep in mind that this is all taking place in the early 1900s in Edwardian England. The Bloomsbury Group not only cast off societal aspersions toward homosexuality, gender roles, and non-monogamy, but the majority of them also went on to create seminal works of art, literature, and intellectual theory. The unconventional community started to dissolve in the 1930s as its core members began to pass away. The creations of the Bloomsbury Group affected other modernist writers of the time, including James Joyce and D. H. Law-rence, both of whom went on to publish scandalously sexual yet groundbreak-ing works of literature.[32]

Other Influential Poly Women:

- Edna St. Vincent Millay (1892–1950)
  Millay's poetry and writings on female sexuality, desire, and feminism earned her recognition and success early in her career; she received the Pulitzer Prize for poetry in 1923.[33] Millay and her husband kept their marriage open for all twenty-six years of their relationship, and she maintained concurrent relationships with both men and women during this time.[34, 35]
- Simone de Beauvoir (1908–1986)
  De Beauvoir was a writer, philosopher, political activist, and feminist. She is best known for writing *The Second Sex,* which became a foundational text for feminist philosophy.[36] The famed philosopher Jean-Paul Sartre proposed marriage to de Beauvoir in 1929, but she refused. Instead, the couple maintained an open relationship for over fifty years, enjoying a number of lovers both together and separately.[37]
- Elizabeth Holloway Marston (1893–1993)
  Marston emphatically broke the mold of women of her time, earning three higher degrees in psychology and law. She and her husband, psychologist Charles Moulton, made groundbreaking research that paved the way for the first lie-detector tests.[38] Marston and her husband lived in a triad relationship with one of his university students, Olive Byrne, and the three raised four children together in their family home. You may not be familiar with this over-achieving trio, but you are most likely familiar with Charles Moulton's beloved creation: Wonder Woman. Moulton based the evil-thwarting Amazonian superheroine and feminist icon on his indomitable wife and mistress.[39]

The 1950s and '60s

After the upheaval of World War II, there was a surge in church attendance and in the rates of marriage and childbirth, particularly in America. The 1950s gave us the image of the perfect housewife—a dutiful mother and submissive wife, faithful, self-sacrificing, and fully devoted to keeping her husband and children happy and well-fed. The subsequent decades would bring a wave of social rebellion and a sexually liberated youth culture seeking to demolish this image. However, the sexual revolution of the sixties actually had its silent beginnings in the conservative fifties.[40]

Alfred Kinsey's reports on the sexual behavior of men and women, released in 1948 and 1953, respectively, caused a huge stir. The reports exposed what was actually happening in the bedroom behind the pure and wholesome facade expected of married couples. Kinsey's studies revealed that the majority of the population had had premarital sex, and that nearly half of men had engaged in both heterosexual and homosexual activities over the course of their lifetime. He also found that 50 percent of men and 26 percent of women had engaged in extramarital affairs.[41] Evangelist Billy Graham embodied the Church's outrage and society's shock at these statistics by stating that Dr. Kinsey "certainly could not have interviewed any of the millions of born-again Christian women in this country who put the highest price on virtue, decency and modesty."[42]

The message was clear: men and women like sex, including sex outside of social norms. However, getting people to actually talk about this fact was an uphill battle until the major cultural shifts of the sixties. The birth control pill hit the market in 1960, and in the fog of a bitter foreign war and heated civil rights movement, attitudes toward marriage, sex, and monogamy were turned on their head.[43]

Swinging and Free Love

The modern-day polyamory movement has its roots in the sexual revolutions of the sixties and seventies, which are characterized by their infamous counterculture movements. Ask people about this time, and you'll find talk of bell bottom-clad hippies preaching the message of pscyhedelics and free love. Others will call to mind extravagant "key parties"—a sensationalized picture of an unrestrained and irresponsible generation of hedonists. Modern-day perceptions of polyamory and non-monogamy are still colored by the precedent laid down by the movement's sexually rebellious forebears, for better or for worse.

The unfortunately named practice of "wife-swapping" started in the fifties, with couples placing clandestine advertisements in the newspaper seeking other couples for sexual play within the privacy of the home. This pastime reached its heyday in the sixties, when an organization in Berkeley, California known as the Sexual Freedom League openly acknowledged the swinging movement.[44] Scientists began seeking to examine swinging couples and performed research studies determining the benefits of the practice. As the swinging scene continued to pick up steam in the eighties, distinct schools of thought began to form. *Recreational swingers*—swingers in a closed relationship who only play in the context of parties and clubs—became distinguished from *utopian swingers*—swingers who develop ongoing connections and friendships with other couples that they play with.[45] Utopian swingers were the forerunners of the modern-day polyamory movement, and there is controversy today over whether this kind of swinging can be categorized as polyamory or not.

During this time, the free love movement was also gaining followers. Feminists decried the institution of marriage as a source of enslavement and subjugation for women. More people began to question the importance of marriage and monogamy, as well as the government's role in policing them. The pill, now more widely available, put the power of reproductive choice back into the hands of women, but this power was not without its price. With the concern of pregnancy struck from the table, women had also lost an effective bargaining chip to say no to unwanted sex. Anecdotal evidence from this time is awash with stories of men pressuring and coercing women into casual sex, with little regard for or basic knowledge of STI prevention. The fact that casual sex approached the borderline of acceptability at all was a far cry from the dominant and conservative attitudes of the 50s, but it took many more years before open discussions on safety, responsibility, and consent entered the picture.

It was in this atmosphere that the some of the first swingers clubs, nudist resorts, and free love intentional communities came to be. For the first time in a very long time, the sexually and romantically deviant could find support networks of kindred spirits. Some of the intentional communities begun at this time are still going strong to this day, and several were paramount in bringing polyamory and ethical non-monogamy to the public eye.

The O'Neills and Open Marriage

Did you know that the term *open marriage* wasn't originally meant for non-monogamous relationships?

In 1972, researchers George and Nena O'Neill published *Open Marriage: A New Lifestyle for Couples*. Their book was a groundbreaking critical look at the expectations for traditional marriage and gender roles. Contrary to popular belief, the O'Neills did not directly encourage couples to have extramarital sex. Rather, their research stressed the importance of examining how stiff cultural expectations were keeping married people unhappy. The O'Neills put forth that open communication, flexibility, an outside support network, and an overall environment that contributed to each person's growth was what made a marriage "open."[46] The O'Neills' book only made brief mention of the possibility of non-monogamy, but for several years after, it became the defining feature of their book in pop culture.

Kerista Commune and Others

The Kerista commune is credited with first coining the term *polyfidelity* to describe a relationship that involved more than two people, but wherein each person committed to only engage romantically and sexually with people inside the relationship.[47] People outside of the relationship are prohibited, except with the consent of each member involved. Polyfidelity was integral to the foundations of the Kerista commune, whose members practiced something that looked very similar to group marriage.

Founded in 1971, the Kerista commune was a radical experiment in utopian, polyamorous living. Members were organized into groups of people referred to as Best Friend Identity Clusters or BFICs. These groups could be as small as four people or as large as twenty-four. Tightly regimented sleeping schedules were rotated so that each member of the BFIC shared a bed with a different member of the opposite sex each night of the week. (Though the Kerista commune supported the efforts for gay rights in its day, it did not encourage its members to partake in any homosexual activity, nor did it offer extensive support toward its members who were bisexual or homosexual.) Each member was tested for STIs regularly, and men were required to undergo a vasectomy. Members of the group were heavily discouraged from giving "preferential treatment" to any one person in their BFIC. If you were not equally attracted to each opposite-sex member of your group, you were eligible to be placed into a different BFIC, or you were invited to bring the issue up during communal "gestalt" sessions, which could run the range from a simple, problem-solving conversation to full-on bullying by other members of the group.[48]

The community lasted over thirty years, finally disbanding due to conflicts over financial management and the rigidity with which relationships were monitored and controlled.[49] As seen in the Oneida Community, the philosophy behind communal polyamorous living was good on paper but ultimately stifled by people in authority attempting to dictate and control the sexual and romantic behavior of others.

The Kerista commune did contribute another word to the polyamory lexicon: *compersion*. Compersion is a hybrid of "compassion" and "conversion," and it describes positive feelings about the happiness your partner experiences with other partners. Essentially, compersion is the opposite of jealousy. Much more on compersion in chapter 8.

Polyamory and Paganism

As the Kerista commune continued to grow during the eighties, another counterculture community was also increasing in visibility: pagans. Neo-paganism, tracing its roots to Old World, animistic spiritual practices, developed in stark contrast to the stiff, restrained tenets of Judeo-Christian religions.[50] Paganism holds sexuality indivisible from divinity, and life energy and erotic energy as a palpable force often used in ritual. The movement's embrace of sex- and body-positivity has drawn feminists, folk from all varieties of sexual identity, and many from the genderqueer and trans populations.[51]

This positive culture also fostered a safe place for practitioners to explore having multiple sexual-loving relationships. In 1990, Morning Glory Zell, a respected Pagan priestess and author, published an article about managing multiple open relationships, describing the people who engage in such a lifestyle as "poly-amorous."[52] The term itself was not new, but it was rapidly adopted as an identifying label and soon morphed from an adjective into a noun: polyamory.

The Internet Age and Cuddle Parties

Morning Glory Zell's debut of the term was perfectly timed. The early nineties saw the nascent stages of Internet use, which was rapidly becoming accessible to the layman, not just the technologically gifted. Bulletin Board Systems (BBS), Usenet groups, and chat rooms may be archaic today, but at the time they were the only places for social networking online. These early networks enabled people to connect as they never had before, giving rise to all kinds of phenomena: open-source information databases, the aggregation of pornography that catered to specific fetishes, and a newfound cohesion among fringe groups, such as those practicing swinging and polyamory.

The word "polyamory" began to show up online, being coined for a second time among Internet users outside of pagan circles.[53] Polyamory support groups began to form, both online and off, and books on non-monogamy began to catch the public eye. Ryam Nearing, while living in a closed triad with her two husbands, published *The Polyfidelity Primer*. Shortly afterward, in 1992, Deborah Anapol published *Polyamory: The New Love Without Limits*.[54] Both works established Nearing and Anapol as key thought-leaders in launching the modern-day polyamory movement. Anapol and Nearing combined their individual networks of polyamorous supporters and practitioners into one by creating the Loving More organization, a nonprofit dedicated to providing education and generating awareness for polyamory and relationship choice.[55] Dossie Easton and Janet Hardy published *The Ethical Slut* in 1997—for many years considered to be the Bible of polyamory and open relationships—which went on to become many people's first exposure to the practicalities of conducting non-monogamous relationships (including mine).

Much of the continuation of the polyamory movement since the nineties has been fueled by the Internet. Websites and blogs devoted to the subject are popping up every day. The advent of social media networks like Facebook, Twitter, and Reddit have allowed non-monogamous people from all walks of life to meet, exchange stories, ask for advice, and share resources. Polyamory meet-ups and workshops range from question-and-answer sessions to *cuddle parties*—people coming together to share nonsexual touch, pajamas optional.[56] News stories, reality shows, and documentaries on non-monogamy are increasing, and alternative relationships are slowly making their way into the realm of public awareness.

Statistics on polyamory and non-monogamy are few and far between; however, with the upswing in awareness, there is an increasing interest in studying and documenting people who engage in these lifestyles. An estimated 4 to 5 percent of the American population openly report being in some kind of consensually non-monogamous relationship, a figure that is still shifting and difficult to pin down.[57] Recall from chapter 1 that even deciding who counts as polyamorous or not is still up in the air. Regardless of statistics, there is undoubtedly a growing tide of curiosity, scandal, acceptance, and discussion surrounding nontraditional love.

Chapter 2 Homework

Exercise #1

Take a moment to think about your family history. Which relationship models have been practiced in your immediate and extended family? Is there a history of unbroken, long-term monogamy? Infidelity? Divorce and remarriage? Polyamory?

Section II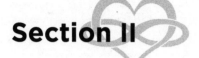

Pre-Reqs

3 *Gnothi Seauton*: How to Know Yourself Inside and Out

Many people will tell you that the most important foundation of any relationship is communication. Indeed, "Communicate, communicate, communicate!" has become the unofficial motto of the polyamorous community. To be fair, effective communication will get you out of most relationship jams, and good communicators will have an easier time in an open relationship. However, there is one quality that is even more important: self-awareness.

The ancient Greeks knew what was up. It was engraved in the wall at the Temple of Apollo at Delphi (which is where the Oracle of Delphi hung out): *Gnothi Seauton.* Know thyself. Although "Gnothi seauton, gnothi seauton, gnothi seauton!" is not quite as catchy as far as mottos go.

Many people spend their entire lives without questioning *why* they are the way they are or *how* they came to be that way. This is perfectly normal. A bear doesn't question why it has a compelling desire to rifle through an unguarded trash can. A fish is not really aware of the water in which it swims, just as we are only peripherally aware of the air and space that surrounds us. But this goes beyond our awareness of physical existence and consciousness. A person can go years without *actually* knowing why she wears makeup every day, why she is constantly running late, why certain people rub her the wrong way, or why she eats eggs and toast for breakfast instead of fish and rice. Instead of examining the *why* and *how*, we're generally pretty content to say, "That's just the way I am."

Self-awareness is the process of bringing the why and how to the surface, and it is a necessary step *before* effective communication. If you know your deep-seated desires, insecurities, beliefs, vulnerabilities, strengths, weaknesses, and triggers, then you can begin envisioning what your ideal romantic life could be. You can begin to illuminate what you need or want out of love, sex, dates, or long-term relationships. You can understand why certain acts and thoughts inspire feelings of jealousy or insecurity or arousal or gratitude.

It is tempting to settle for surface-level self-awareness. "That's just the way I am" gets you off the hook and frees you from having to challenge or question any part of yourself. If you really dig in to who you are and what makes you tick, you'll probably be surprised to discover that there is no *one* way that you are. The desires, emotions, impulses, and fears that make up your psyche are never static. They are constantly shifting depending on your environment, your circumstances, your age, or what kind of day at work you had. One moment is jealousy, the next is peace, the next is compersion, the next is fear, then it comes back around to jealousy, then to gratitude, and so on and so forth. Claiming "I am a jealous person" or "I am a peaceful person" or "I am a nervous person" is simultaneously true and false. Having the ability to clearly see within and observe the changing landscape inside is paramount when embarking on the vulnerable journey of pursuing healthy relationships.

This process is also known as *deconstruction*, which doesn't exactly sound pleasant. Most of us are quite happy to go through our days feeling sturdily constructed, thank you very much. The path to deconstructed self-awareness is also riddled with embarrassing stumbling blocks. You will make mistakes in communication, and you will be the victim of other people's mistakes. Unexpected flare-ups of anger or jealousy will be painful lessons about your triggers and insecurities. As you peel away your layers, strange and uncomfortable facets of yourself may be revealed. But the wisdom, growth, and power you will gain is priceless.

This chapter presents a number of self-inquiry questions and points to consider about love, relationships, sex, fears, and more. It can be useful to write down your answers to these questions. It can also be insightful to share your answers with a partner, family member, or friend, and to hear their responses as well. Some of these inquiries might be a little too heavy-hitting for a first date, but I won't stop you if you're wanting to get very up close and personal with someone from the get-go.

Another great thing about self-awareness is that it can be obtained by any number of means, not just by using the questions in this chapter. Meditation, self-development courses or books, spiritual practice, therapy, or any other kind of courageous self-examination can put you on the right track, and those will be covered in more detail later on.

I Believe in a Thing Called Love

Deconstructing love is no easy task. On the one hand, you can take the clinical route and observe love as merely a cocktail of brain chemicals that explodes your body into reproduction mode when it encounters someone who has healthy-smelling pheromones and appears to be of good breeding stock. You may find this approach to be too dry and better suited to the world of animal husbandry. Or, if you're a left-brained lover of logic, this may be the perfect definition. On the other hand, you can take the idealistic viewpoint and rejoice in love being an all-powerful force of rainbow magic capable of healing the world, curing cancer, and even making Shakespearean double suicide romantic. This view might fill you with warm fuzzies, or it might be a little too mushy and sentimental for your tastes.

As I've undertaken years of introspection and observed myself in love, I've found that my personal definition of love leans more left-brained in acknowledging its chemical and biological influence, with just the right amount of mushiness mixed in for flavor. This approach has helped me maintain perspective and keep my feet on the ground while being tossed around in the drunken tailspin that is falling in love with someone new. It's also allowed me to soak in those indescribable moments where I can see a partner at his or her worst—sick, tired, vulnerable, or depressed—and still somehow feel an unfathomable depth of love and care.

Your personal definition of love is also characterized by how you look at the difference between *loving* someone and *falling in love* with someone. The intense, intoxicating, head-over-heels feelings you get when falling in love do not generally last throughout the course of a long-term relationship. Excitement fades, bonding grows, and as much as you love your partner, the butterflies don't stick around.

That may sound like it comes from the files of Captain Obvious, but there are countless magazine articles, advice columns, and even entire books devoted to bringing the "spark" back to a relationship. Society applauds couples who have managed to stay married for decades (happily or not), and everyone is always dying to know what their secret is. So many monogamous couples undergo feelings of frustration when the affection, flirtation, cuddling, and sex is not the same ten years into the relationship as it was at the beginning.

Part of this is symptomatic of our cultural obsession with finding "The One" or "Mr. Right." The unspoken implication is that if you're actually with the right person, those butterflies won't fade, the sex will be just as hot as it was on day one, and no one will ever get remotely bored. The other part is linked to the universal fear of change. When we experience something so thrilling, so tasty, so damn *good* as falling in love, we don't want it to go away, and we don't want it to change into something else.

Like all of existence, love changes all the time, *and that's okay.* On a practical, biological level, your brain just can't keep up with the amount of love drugs it's required to pump out in order to keep you in that lovesick high all the time. Outside of that, the falling–in–love fuzzies need to change in order for you to experience other kinds of love. Much the same way as people living in icy environments coin dozens of words for the different types of snow, there are so many different and wonderful kinds of love, though we have yet to develop the vocabulary for it. There's the love that comes from sharing a collection of inside jokes with someone. There's the love that comes from a partner telling you that you're sexy even when you're un–showered and not wearing makeup. There's the love that comes from the first time you let yourself cry in front of someone. And so many more than that.

Of course, one of the great benefits of polyamory is that you can experience the let's-cuddle-and-eat-junk-food-and-binge-watch-Netflix-all-day kind of love and the flirty-fluttery-hot-date-huge-crush kind of love at the same time. Neither form of love is more important or more valid than the other. It's kind of like having your cake, eating it too, and licking the frosting off the plate afterward.

Take this time to check in with yourself and what your expectations are for the changing tide that is love. Whether your experience of love is more art or more science, it is important to examine your personal outlook on love, how you respond when falling in love, and how that affects the way you approach relationships. Gaining this kind of self-awareness is the first step in learning how to approach love and new relationships in a way that keeps your feet on the ground and your head on your shoulders, but with your heart still getting to soar through the air. Here are some questions to get you started:

- *How do you know when you have fallen in love? How do you know when it's time to say "I love you" to your partner?*
- *What is it that you like about falling in love? What are the physical sensations you experience when you're in love?*

- *How do you know when someone loves you? What do you need to see/hear/feel in order to believe that someone loves you?*
- *Have you made any life decisions (e.g. moving to a new city, quitting or changing jobs, ending another relationship or friendship) while falling in love? When those feelings faded, which decisions did you regret? Which decisions were you still happy with?*
- *How do you feel about the idea of finding a soul mate? Which do you find to be more romantic: having one soul mate, or multiple soul mates?*
- *Do you rarely experience romantic feelings or sexual attraction for other people?* (If this is you, you can read more on aromanticism and asexuality in chapter 6.)

Like a Horse and Carriage

The old Frank Sinatra song says that love and marriage go together like a horse and carriage. It's true that modern-day marriage (or any long-term relationship) is usually intertwined with love, but the two are very different entities. If the song is to be believed, one of them is a rearing, bucking, snorting, two-thousand-pound beast, but I'll leave it up to your own interpretation to decide which one is which.

Reconciling the lofty, ideal nature of love and the everyday, all-too-real nature of interpersonal relationships is a never-ending quest. How do you square loving your partner wholeheartedly and giving her your best self while also having to ask her for the *billionth* time to load the dishwasher correctly? How do you trust that your partner is filled with adoration and attraction for you, even though he wakes up every morning to see you conked out with drool all over the pillow and hair like David Bowie in *The Labyrinth*? How do you create relationships that perfectly blend the real with the ideal?

The Relationship Escalator

Your expectations for relationships may be heavily influenced by the culturally bolstered importance of the *relationship escalator*. The relationship escalator is the belief that a relationship is not legitimate unless it is following the standard upward trajectory: dating > sex > exclusivity > moving in together > marriage > kids > 'til death do us part. There is a deeply ingrained expectation that if a relationship is truly "serious," it will automatically lead to these things.[1] Once when I was sharing with a family member how happy I was that my new partner shared my relationship values, which included not tying the knot, she was flabbergasted and asked, "If you don't want to get married, what's the point of the relationship?"

The relationship escalator can turn regular dating into a total nightmare. If you know that any relationship you begin is expected to run the full course of the escalator, there's incredible pressure to pick the right person. Dates can end up feeling less like a fun social outing and more like a future spouse audition.

When you open up your heart to multiple partners, it changes the game. It requires you to step off of the escalator and let each individual relationship find its own path organically. If you're someone like me, who doesn't have a strong desire to get legally married, it forces you to evaluate the shape you want your relationships to take and how you want to negotiate long-term partnerships outside of a marriage contract. (Although those tax breaks are mighty tempting.)

For example, one of my partners a few years back was a man who worked a ridiculously demanding job. Our chemistry was amazing, and our dates together consisted of hours of intellectual conversation, enjoying quality wine, and voracious love-making. However, his job schedule only allowed us to see each other once a week, and only from the hours of 10 p.m. to 8 a.m. Had I entered this relationship expecting him to follow me up the relationship escalator, I would have gotten frustrated and disappointed very quickly. In allowing the relationship to reach its own level, we were able to enjoy a long-lasting connection that enhanced each other's lives without adding pressure or forcing it to be something it could not be within those circumstances.

This does not mean that the individual events that make up the relationship escalator are bad. You may still like the idea of making a long-term, loving commitment, raising children of your own, or growing old together. But those events don't all have to happen in the same relationship. Or they could happen in multiple relationships! You've already determined your thoughts and feelings about love; now it's time to observe your feelings about relationships. Try the following questions:

- *What do you like about romantic relationships? What do you expect to happen when you start a new relationship?*
- *What do you dislike about romantic relationships? What are the things that you're afraid of when you start a new relationship?*
- *How do your relationships usually begin? Do you tend to go for a slow burn or do you engage very quickly and passionately?*

- *How do your relationships usually end? Is there any kind of recurring pattern (both positive and negative) in your history of relationships?*
- *What are the best personal qualities that you bring to a relationship? What have current or past partners appreciated about you?*
- *Which parts of the relationship escalator do you want in your life? Which parts could you do without?*
- *What is your history with monogamy? Has it been a struggle, or has it been easy for you?*

Divided by a Common Language

Until "Gnothi seauton, gnothi seauton, gnothi seauton!" spreads like wildfire, the go-to slogan for alternative relationships remains "Communicate, communicate, communicate!" The necessity of communication is a no-brainer, but why is it so easy to mess it up? Over the course of many years of being in poly relationships, my communication skills have by necessity skyrocketed, but I *still* have trouble with it on a daily basis. You'll find tactics for building communication skills and methods for tackling difficult conversations in chapter 4, but first, determine what kind of communication habits you're bringing to the table.

Communication patterns are impressed on us from a young age. Our parents and other primary adult figures around us set the tone for socializing and conflict resolution that many of us end up carrying into our adult lives. Often these habits are a mix of healthy and unhealthy, effective and dysfunctional. Rarely does anyone make it out of childhood without at least a few communication neuroses. You may be totally stunted and awkward when it comes to expressing positive emotions to your partners, but excel at sharing your negative emotions and fears in a proactive and nonconfrontational way. Or you may be the exact opposite. Your particular communication style can and will come up in every interpersonal relationship you have, so it's important to gain awareness of it.

Spewers and Chewers

In the course of my time examining myself and my partners and helping many clients through the ups and downs of communication, I've found that people tend to fall into two categories when communicating the bulk of their thoughts, feelings, and opinions. Two categories may seem reductive, but of course there are many gradients and unique styles within the two. The highly scientific labels I've attached to these two categories are *spewers* and *chewers*.

Spewers don't like to have things on their chest. Whether they are bursting with ooey-gooey, lovey-dovey feelings or they're trembling with rage, they're likely to let you know about it sooner rather than later. Spewers have a strong need to talk out their emotions or to vent their feelings. Verbally "spewing" it all out releases the pressure of built-up emotions, which frees up their energy to focus clearly on whatever the next step should be.

Chewers, on the other hand, keep their cards closer to the vest. When emotion arises, they are generally tight-lipped, preferring to mull over the circumstances and their own thoughts and feelings before expressing anything. Chewers tend to focus on how to say the *right* thing and will refrain from saying too much before they've figured out exactly how it should be said. They feel much more comfortable proceeding in communication or problem-solving once they've spent the requisite time "chewing" on their thoughts and getting them organized.

Spewers and chewers are capable of having harmonious communication within their relationship, provided they understand each other. I'm a chewer myself, and I have had to learn not only how to proactively ask for space and time for chewing, but also ways to reassure my partner that I'm not checking out or avoiding communication entirely. I've also needed to learn how to give my partners who are spewers a safe space to effectively vent their feelings without judgment and without taking it personally.

Love Languages

In the bestselling book *The Five Love Languages,* author Gary D. Chapman categorizes five different ways that people express love to their partner and prefer to receive love from their partner. When you are fluent in your partner's love language, you can know for sure that your expressions of love, appreciation, and security are hitting their mark. Chapman's five love languages are:

- Words of Affirmation
- Quality Time
- Receiving Gifts
- Acts of Service
- Physical Touch

You can evaluate your love language by taking a handy quiz at *5lovelanguages.com.*

The Best Policy

Polyamory requires blunt, transparent honesty about one's innermost feelings, thoughts, fears, and desires. Ironically, most of us have been culturally taught that romantic relationships are no place for this level of honesty. If you're attracted to a person other than your partner, you'd better keep it to yourself. Should you go so far as to be affectionate or sexual with an outside party, there is no way in hell that information can be revealed without causing major destruction. That's accepted as common sense.

Yet ethically non-monogamous relationships require the exact opposite of this kind of common sense. It is a requirement that you be honest with your partners from the get-go that your intention is to be non-monogamous, as well as being up-front about how many partners you have. It is absolutely necessary to be transparent about your safe sex practices, and about your sexual health. If you're feeling insecure or vulnerable, it is crucial to reveal your feelings instead of hiding behind the facade of "I'm fine." This doesn't mean you have to divulge every minutia of your sex life with one partner to all of your other partners, nor does it mean that no one gets to have any privacy. But it does mean that your partners should be able to trust that you are providing them with necessary information truthfully and proactively.

Just like communication patterns, our relationship to honesty and transparency begins at a very early age. One of my clients, Mark, was in an open marriage but having a lot of difficulty being fully transparent with his wife about his other relationships. Even though both had agreed that having other partners was okay, Mark still found himself hiding details of how often he had seen someone and how intimate his relationships were. The omissions were causing immense amounts of strain in the relationship, even though they had been happily non-monogamous for years.

After therapy, intense personal work, and self-inquiry, Mark realized that his ineffective relationship with honesty was established in his childhood. He grew up with an abusive father, and whenever Mark made a mistake at school or at home, his father would beat him. From a young age, Mark got in the habit of omitting information and making elaborate cover-ups—if he accidentally broke a toy or a tool, he buried it in the backyard. This habit carried over to his adult life, even in the context of a non-abusive relationship.

Once Mark was finally aware of this well-worn neural pathway, he had the ability to get in front of it. Knowing that his habit was to omit information out of fear, he was able to ask his wife for reassurance that nothing bad would happen if he shared information openly and honestly. If being blatantly honest with your partners makes you feel uneasy or anxious, or if you find yourself resorting to omitting information, it can be helpful to examine what kind of relationship to honesty was established when you were young. If you're aware of patterns and habits established long ago, you can gain the power to begin reshaping them, as Mark did.

Fighting Words

Believe it or not, you will not agree with your romantic partner 100 percent of the time. Increase the number of partners you have, and you increase the likelihood that *someone* is going to disagree with *somebody* at *some* point. Arguments are no one's favorite pastime, but peaceful relationships require potent conflict resolution skills. Everyone has their own totally unique style of handling conflict. Over the course of our lives we learn how to fight (fairly or unfairly) from arguments with parents, siblings, friends, and past lovers.

When unpleasant conversations arise, stress hormones are triggered as part of the fight-or-flight response. This doesn't mean that you're actually getting ready to box your boyfriend's ears, or to go cower behind the couch (provided your relationship is healthy and non-abusive). But in arguments, each of us has a set of go-to mental moves for offense, defense, and retreat. When you are *sure* that you're right and the other person is wrong, what do you do? If your sparring partner is gaining the upper hand, how do you react? If someone verbally attacks you, what's your go-to to get them off your back?

Under the stress of a fight, people do all sorts of things—resorting to insults (direct or implied), digging up the other person's past faults, belittling and mocking, shutting down, giving the silent treatment, walking away and slamming the door, being a martyr, the list goes on. I've gotten particularly adept at a strategy I like to call "Concede Your Way to Victory." The ol' CYWTV technique involves a lot of saying, "Okay, fine, you win. You're right. Do whatever you want to do," and then sulking icily until the other person feels bad enough to be the first to apologize. It ain't pretty.

It's hard to be on your best, most angelic behavior when emotions are running high. When the stakes are high (the person you love thinking that you're wrong can feel pretty high-stakes), all too often we sacrifice real communication in favor of being right. That's where the verbal parries, the strategies, the games creep in. At some point in my past, the CYWTV technique must have worked—not for actual communication, but for making me right and the other person wrong. When it first worked, it must have felt really good, because it's managed to make its way back into many, many arguments since then. This is how we find ourselves having the same argument with the same person over and over again. Topics and circumstances change, but rarely do we examine what's in our mental arsenal, or question why we're hoarding those weapons in the first place.

This is the time to peek into the inner weapons rack. When you know how your fight-or-flight response affects the way you argue, you no longer have to be ruled by it. It's the first step to forming new, positive communication habits for resolving conflict (which you'll learn more about in chapter 4). If you're under the impression that you *don't* have a particular way you fight or that you *don't* resort to a myriad of strategies to make yourself right and the other person wrong, go ask someone who has been in an argument with you at least three times (parents, siblings, and exes are great for this). Prepare for an uncomfortable but highly enlightening conversation.

- *What patterns for communication and conflict resolution did you see growing up? Have you seen those patterns mirrored in your romantic relationships?*
- *Are you a chewer or a spewer? Are there certain topics where you're more comfortable being a chewer or a spewer?*
- *How do you handle honesty? Are you an open book, or do you prefer to keep things to yourself? Is it easy or difficult for you to lie to someone?*
- *How do you express love to your romantic partners? What kind of love language do you prefer to receive from your romantic partners?*
- *What is your communication style in arguments? What strategies do you employ to make yourself right and the other person wrong?*
- *When you're getting emotional in an argument, how do you manage it? Is it easy for you to walk away to cool off, or do you need to hash it all out right in the moment?*

Sex and Sexuality

This book is not a sex manual (there are hundreds of other books out there doing a much better job of that). In chapter 6, you will find information about expressing sexual needs, defining your boundaries, exploring the spectrum of your own sexuality, and navigating the logistics of multi-partner sexual encounters. But in this section, it's time to take stock of your sexy side.

People who do not choose to pursue lifelong heterosexual monogamy are often misrepresented as a bunch of irresponsible, sex-addicted ne'er-do-wells hell-bent on ruining the institution of marriage and family. Because of the looming social stigma, many longtime practitioners of ethical non-monogamy will de-emphasize the role that sex plays in their relationships. Countless bloggers, public speakers, and activists are quick to assure the media, their audiences, and their family and friends that polyamory is *not* all about sex.

But despite desperate attempts to downplay the "dark side," sex is a significant part of our existence. You wouldn't be here without it. It is one of our oldest forms of social bonding and a deeply rooted instinct. Sex is part of our psychology, and that means it also causes some troubling questions. *Am I sexy enough? Do I think about sex too much? Is my sex drive too high? Too low?* For women, there's the added stress of worrying about pregnancy, about being labeled as "frigid" if you don't want to have sex, or being labeled as "slutty" if you do. If you're a woman who is vocal about enjoying sex, or about desiring sex with multiple partners, it won't be long before you realize how hard it is to escape this cultural conditioning.

Our primal sex drives also allow us to find transcendent joy in intimate lovemaking, in creating life, in sharing playful pleasure with others. That's the side of sex that lights us up and connects us more deeply to others. That's the earth-shattering side of sex that fuels *sex positivity.*

Sex positivity does not necessarily mean that all forms of sex are inherently good and must be enthusiastically embraced, but it does encourage breaking out of the old paradigms that say sex is wrong, sinful, dirty, or unhealthy. It's abandoning the notion that a sexually active woman is loose, used up, or morally inferior. It's seeking to actively educate yourself about sexual health and safe sex instead of relying on sensationalized information from the media, your high school health class, or gossip from your friends. It's embracing sex in its multitude of forms, having the open-mindedness to try new things, and being levelheaded enough to know yourself and your boundaries.

You do not have to be sexually active or in any kind of sexual relationship in order to be sex positive. You may already be gung-ho about all of this, or you may still feel hesitant or awkward thinking and talking about sex. Maybe you were raised in a sex-positive environment, or maybe sex positivity is difficult for you because of a history of abuse or negative attitudes imposed by your parents. Either way, check in with yourself and get curious about what kind of sexual being you are and what kind of thoughts, feelings, and opinions about sex you may have.

- *What role has sex played in your life and in your past relationships?*
- *Which kinds of sex do you enjoy and fantasize about? Which kinds of sex scare you or intimidate you?*
- *Do you ever feel ashamed about your sex drive being too low or too high?*
- *Do you require sex in every romantic relationship?*
- *Is there a particular type of sex/frequency of sex you've always wanted but have never gotten in your past relationships?*
- *Is there a type of sex that you want, but are too ashamed or embarrassed to ask anybody?*
- *Is it difficult for you to share sexual fantasies or desires with a partner? What about talking about sexual history?*
- *What has been your primary source of knowledge about STIs and safe sex?*
- *What are your boundaries when it comes to practicing safe sex? What level of risk are you comfortable with?* (There will be more on this in chapter 6.)

The Fluidity of Sexuality

Answering some of these questions about sex may have brought up thoughts or questions about your sexuality or gender identity. That's a whole other part of yourself to discover if you haven't already! The spectrum of your own sexuality may be hitherto unexplored and unquestioned, or you may have already spent a lot of time inquiring, exploring, and experimenting to figure out exactly who or what makes you tick and gets you excited. Many people find polyamorous and non-monogamous relationships to be a safe place to explore outside their edges of sexuality and gender. This may include finding acceptance if you are exploring gender non-conformity. See chapter 6 for more discussion on sexuality and gender.

Fears and Insecurities

The very concept of being in a relationship where you're "sharing" a partner with multiple others is abjectly terrifying to many. No one enjoys feeling jealous, and the default tactic is to make sure to avoid jealousy-causing circumstances at all costs. To some people this means making sure your partner doesn't hang out with any attractive coworkers, never speaks to his ex-girlfriend, and never checks out anyone else. Within non-monogamous relationships, this shows up in the form of never wanting to hear any details about your partner's other partners, or setting up restrictions on how intimate other relationships can grow. Chapter 7 has a whole list of common strategies for solving jealousy that don't actually solve anything.

The problem is that these behaviors treat the symptom but not the disease. Jealousy is a complex emotion, and the heart of it is wrapped up in our own fears and insecurities. It's a common mistake to think that if your partner is kind enough, loves you enough, communicates enough, just *is enough*, then all your doubts will disappear. Unfortunately, relationships don't always work that way, even healthy ones.

Relationships are a strange paradox. We need the human connection and support that relationships of every kind provide. The fear of being alone is universal. Yet relationships themselves rarely allay our fears or insecurities. If anything, we sometimes get even more afraid and insecure—that the other person will find us unattractive, will get bored, will leave. Even when we're not alone, we are still afraid of being alone.

The fear of losing a partner and being alone manifests in many ways: jealousy, anger, anxiety, possessiveness, competition, arrogance, indifference, and many other unsavory attitudes. The irony is that all of these are great tactics for driving a partner away. The tighter you squeeze someone you love, the easier it is for them to slip through your fingers.

No amount of reassurance from someone else can change the negative opinions you hold about yourself. If you deeply believe that your tummy is a shameful piece of disgusting flab, that belief will not change after your partner says "You're sexy!" for the thirty-seventh time. It is important to figure out now what these deeply held negative beliefs are. It can be unpleasant, but here is the place to dig deep and examine the small, scared part of you without judgment. Discovering your vulnerabilities gives you an opportunity to be gentle with yourself and enables you to give your partners insights into the things that trigger your jealousies and anxieties.

- *What is your deepest fear regarding love and sex?*
- *If you're new to polyamory or non-monogamy, what scares you about it?*
- *What parts of yourself and your life (your body, your career, your bank account, etc.) are you most insecure about?*
- *What parts of yourself and your life are you most proud of?*
- *What does jealousy feel like to you? What are the physical sensations that you feel when you're jealous?*
- *When you are jealous of a coworker, family member, or friend, how do you cope with it?*
- *When you are jealous within a romantic relationship, how do you cope with it?*

Your Relationship Vision

If you picked up this book, it's likely you are interested in approaching relationships differently. Maybe monogamy failed you in the past, maybe you've been curious about alternative relationships for a long time, or maybe you love doing anything that's out of the mainstream. (Perhaps someday a few of us can sprout ironic mustaches and proclaim, "I was into polyamory *before* it was cool!") Regardless of your reasons, you're someone who is ready to stop playing by someone else's rules.

That's easier said than done. Each of us came into the world and were all but handed the exact script for how relationships are supposed to go, what love is supposed to look like, and what we are supposed to want for our love lives. Throwing the script out the window is downright crazy.

But the most exciting thing is . . . you get to write your own script! When you take charge of how you want your love life to look, it's a rare opportunity to start from scratch. Your future decisions don't need to be dictated by the expectations of your family, your culture, your church, or your peer group. Instead, the future of your love life can be a blank canvas, ready for you to start creating a unique masterpiece (or ready for you to go to town on it with finger paints, if that's your style).

After going through the wringer of examining your thoughts, feelings, neuroses, hang-ups, and everything else bouncing around in your psyche, here is the space to have a little fun. If you could really have whatever you wanted in regard to love, sex, and relationships, what would it look like?

Asking that question within the limitless expanse of your mental fantasy land can produce some extreme results—maybe your mind conjures up a harem of Adonises, all scantily clad, oiled up, and ready to compliment your booty. Or perhaps the mental magic wand materializes the girlfriend you've always dreamed of—great in bed, head-turning looks, and happens to also be a millionaire generous enough to spoil you rotten. Or perhaps you envision a large, happy family of partners and metamours (your partners' other partners) dedicated to raising a whole passel of little kids together.

These fantasies may be silly or reasonable, but they are a window into the answer to the next question: If you were to actually have your fantasy life, how would it make you feel? A collection of manly love-servants may not be realistic, but feeling loved, sexually satisfied, and cared for is attainable. Perfect millionaire girlfriends are few and far between, but feeling attraction to a partner who is attentive to your needs is a viable dream. And getting a bunch of adults together to raise a kid? It really does take a village. The village may as well love and care for one another.

As you go through the questions below and continue reading this book, keep in mind that your fantasy love life may be more achievable than you think, though it may not look exactly the way you initially envision it. In the meantime, throw out everything you know about the way relationships are supposed to go, and start crafting the blueprints of the relationships you've always wanted.

- *If you were to close your eyes and wave a magic wand, what would your romantic life look like? What would a perfect relationship (or multiple perfect relationships) look like? Be bold, be vulnerable, be silly, be honest!*
- *If you were to have exactly what you wanted for your love life and sex life, how would it make you feel? How would the people involved with you feel?*
- *What kind of person do you have to be in order to get the love life that you want?*
- *What kind of people do you want to be romantically and sexually involved with?*
- *When you're considering beginning a relationship with someone, what is a deal breaker?*

- *How do you personally define commitment? How do you know if someone is in a committed relationship with you?*
- *If you're interested in monogamy, why is that? What are your reasons for pursuing it?*
- *If you're interested in polyamory or some other form of non-monogamy, why is that? What are your reasons for pursuing it?*
- *What are your thoughts on raising children within your romantic relationships? Would you want just one partner to act as coparent, or could you envision multiple partners raising your children? Would you feel happy being part of the child-rearing process for a child who was not biologically yours?*

Never-ending Journey

Now that you're at the end of the chapter, you should have gotten an amusing, perhaps frightening, and illuminating glimpse into the things that make you tick. However, the journey of self-discovery is never-ending. As you continue to read this book, refer back to your answers from this section. You may be surprised by thoughts that are more fluid and flexible, and you will also see which beliefs are steadfast.

There is so much more you can do for self-awareness beyond the questions in this chapter. Maintain a constant state of curiosity about yourself. When you're in the middle of an angry blowup, or a crying jag, or a fit of laughter, or a puddle of depression, step outside of yourself for just a second and get curious about the intricate universe that is in motion within you.

If you're interested in taking self-awareness to the next level, beyond sex and relationships, check out the Resources section in the back of the book. There is a wealth of information on meditation, therapy, personal development, and more.

Chapter 3 Homework

Exercise #1

Sit down with a friend, lover, family member, or anyone else you're interested in getting to know a *lot* better and ask them the questions above. Share your answers as well.

Exercise #2

Look back over your responses. If you were to answer these questions five years ago, which responses would be vastly different? Which responses would be the same? Which values or aspects of your personality appear to be fixed, and which ones appear to be more fluid?

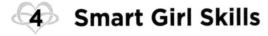

4 Smart Girl Skills

You ever notice that there are some fundamental things they never taught you at school?

For instance, personal finance. Sure, you probably had to learn algebra, calculate percentages, and solve word problems having to do with money. But the standard American education is surprisingly lacking in teaching kids how to actually handle money. Unless your parents were proactive in teaching you, learning the difference between what a credit card's interest rate is versus what it feels like to actually have to pay it was mostly likely a rude wake-up call. It's one thing to know how to calculate 10 percent of your income; it's another thing altogether to develop the diligence to put that 10 percent into your savings every month.

In the same way, the traditional education system does not teach us much about adult relationships. The closest we get are sex ed classes, and even those are hit or miss. Depending on what school district you grew up in, you may have been taught that abstinence until marriage is the only safe way to go, or you may have been traumatized by graphic pictures of extreme cases of untreated STIs. You may have been taught that heterosexual monogamy is the only way to go, or that it's bad to feel like your gender is different from the one printed on your birth certificate. Regardless, most of us didn't get much info on how to conduct a healthy relationship, outside of being told to wear a condom.

We fumble around as teenagers and young adults, making mistakes, experimenting, forming all kinds of habits and approaches to relationships and sex, for better or worse. This extends into later adult years as well, with many people (usually post-divorce) jokingly referring to their first marriage as a "starter marriage" or "practice marriage." We have a bare-bones understanding that relationships are something you can get better at over time, but at the cost of undergoing many failed relationships along the way.

We learn many lessons about communication, compassion, and ourselves from the successes and failures of our relationships. Human relationships help us further these skills, yet having these skills in the first place is what enables our relationships to grow at all. It's a symbiosis. How wonderful would it be to come to a relationship already equipped with the skills to pay the bills, as it were? How excellent would it be to also be in relationships where those skills could continue to be nurtured, helping everyone involved continue to grow and evolve into bad-ass, interpersonally adroit super-humans?

Though some people take to non-monogamous relationships like a fish to water, most people make a lot of mistakes when they first start. Gaining experience and getting "good" at open relationships generally comes with a long history of trial and error, making lots of mistakes, and consciously keeping in mind lessons from the past.

You may be a natural at some of the personal skills discussed in this chapter, and others may take conscious effort and repeated practice before they become second nature. For those skills that do require some work, it's important to keep your eyes on the prize, so to speak. Getting up at 6 a.m. to go for a run is a less than pleasant experience, but your desire to break a new record in your next marathon is what gets you out of bed. If you struggle and hit snags along your personal path of growth, it's useful to have a motivating force in mind. It might be the desire to have more deeply connected and long-lasting relationships, or maybe a wish for inner peace and happiness regardless of circumstances.

Whatever keeps you going when the going gets tough, it's not a requirement to stumble on every pothole in the road to learn what it takes to have relationships that are healthy and successful. After several years of experience in my own poly relationships, witnessing others' relationships, and making an embarrassing number of mistakes, I've found a certain number of personal skills to be prevalent in those relationships that were the happiest. I originally wrote this for Multiamory.com as "7 Habits of Highly Effective Poly Relationships," and to this day it's still one of the site's most popular articles. (There are far more than seven, but Internet audiences just love short, numbered lists.)

You are committed to your partners and to yourself.

Committed? Doesn't that mean marriage? Sexual exclusivity? Sticking to just one partner?

The traditional definition of "commitment" includes all of these things, but when you start breaking out of the traditional mold, it takes on a different meaning.

Your sense of commitment to your partners involves a dedication to being the best possible version of yourself that you can be, and maintaining the responsibility of caring for your partners. When things get tough or feel uncomfortable, your first move isn't to turn tail and head for the hills. Feeling committed and communicating it to your partners is absolutely necessary to engender trust and a sense of stability. It allows you and your partners to live in a realm where communicating with vulnerability is welcomed. It may sound strange, but it's maintaining a sense of fidelity to your relationships, even though there isn't sexual exclusivity.

You also need to stay committed to yourself. This means knowing how to set personal boundaries and learning how to best take care of yourself emotionally, mentally, and physically. Of course you want to collaborate with your partners and make sure everyone is getting what they need, but a commitment to yourself means not letting someone else bully you into doing something you don't want to do or agreeing to a relationship structure that makes you unhappy. You can find more about setting your boundaries in chapter 7.

One of my personal commitments is a commitment to be continually seeking self-improvement, especially when it comes to communication and emotional health. My commitment to my own self-improvement comes in handy when I find myself slipping into unhealthy behavior such as lashing out in anger or being passive–aggressive.

Lastly, this also means having a sense of commitment to polyamory or non-monogamy itself. If you have found that nontraditional relationships are what you want in your life, boldly commit to that choice. If you're still not sure if polyamory is something you want for the rest of your life, it's still more empowering to say to people, "I'm committed to doing this for now and seeing if it's for me," rather than hemming and hawing about it.

"Be honest with yourself, because I don't truly believe there is such a thing as "trying out polyamory." Being poly is about love and even though love sometimes comes with sex, it doesn't have to, and ultimately it is about deep emotional connections. Those are not things that should be entered into lightly.**"** —Theresa

You're ready to talk. And talk more. And talk even more.

If you're considering a nontraditional relationship, be prepared to talk much more than you are probably used to talking about relationships. In reality, all serious relationships (monogamous, polyamorous, or otherwise) require in-depth discussions about boundaries, feelings, needs, and so on. Unfortunately, a lot of us are used to going into relationships on autopilot, expecting that our partner is on the same page. I've run into many unexpected arguments and even seen relationships end because of these kind of assumptions. I'm of the mind that there is no such thing as communicating too clearly, regardless of the subject. It is better to have a partner say, "Yes, I get it. You've told me twice already," than say, "I had no idea you felt that way! Why didn't you tell me?!"

Communication is that all-important skill touted as the key to successful relationships. It's a skill that I've really had to grind away at in order to improve. I've never been much of a talker (chewer here), and I dream of an alternate reality in which most communication happens via interpretive dance instead of talking. It would be so much easier! My struggle has been getting myself to talk more proactively. On the opposite side, I've been with many partners who have the gift of gab (love those spewers). For the people to whom talking comes naturally, it can be important to clarify which things are important to communicate to a partner and which things are part of their verbal processing or "thinking out loud." Whatever your communication style, there are four components to effective communication: knowing *what* to say, knowing *when* to say it, knowing *how* to say it, and, arguably the most important one, *listening*.

What to Say

If you are feeling upset, jealous, confused, neglected, or a mix of all of those, don't tell your partner, "I'm fine." Maintain vigilance of your emotions, take ownership of them, and when it's time to communicate, express your feelings honestly. Sarah Mirk, author of *Sex From Scratch*, said it best: "Honesty over harmony."

Expressing your feelings honestly calls for *emotional responsibility*. That means owning your feelings or, as some have colorfully put it, "holding your own mud." When you're feeling upset, it can be all too easy to say to your partner, "*You* made me jealous/angry/uncomfortable." If you're in a healthy relationship, it is unlikely that your partner did anything to directly spite you, hurt you, or intentionally make you upset. Your emotional state, while influenced by external events and outside factors, is entirely shaped by your internal decisions about how to react in any given moment. In reality, it's more accurate to say, "X happened, and I got jealous/angry/uncomfortable." It's a subtle shift in psychology—it may be your partner's mistake, but it's *your* reaction.

Owning your fears of being alone or admitting that you're feeling threatened by your partner's new crush is not easy. However, being proactively vulnerable to your partner is an excellent way to deepen intimacy and to give your partner the opportunity to offer reassurance. Most of our fears surrounding abandonment or being replaced by another are completely irrational, but human beings are not rational 100 percent of the time. Understand that rationality is almost never at play when it comes to your deepest fears, and take it easy on yourself and on your partner when sharing.

These are the important things to communicate, but most of us totally suck at communicating them, especially when we let our emotions, personal agendas, or desire to be "right" get in the way. That's why it's important to know when and how to communicate these things so that they'll be transmitted and received clearly, effectively, and calmly.

When to Say It

Because communication is a delicate thing, prone to misunderstanding, assumptions, and every variety of lost-in-translation mishap, it is crucial to create the best possible environment to foster effective communication. It's akin to making sure you have the right soil, the correct ratio of sunlight to shade, and a hearty irrigation system in place before planting your garden. Weeds, storms, frost, and hungry gophers will show up, but you can handle anything with a solid environment as your base.

So what does that mean in not-garden terms? If you have found yourself in a communication breakdown with your partner, check in with how you are feeling. Knowing when to H.A.L.T. has merit. Are you feeling hungry, angry, lonely, or tired? If so, right now is probably not the best time to talk, especially if the subject matter is uncomfortable or difficult. If you're hungry, that's an obvious fix. If you're tired, it might be deciding to take a break to take a nap or agreeing to resume discussion in the morning after a full night's rest. But what about feeling angry and lonely? Sometimes those feelings are the very reason you feel you need to talk!

When your negative emotions are stirring, it takes willpower to remain calm and respectful when hashing things out with your partner. However, your willpower is a limited resource, and trying to stuff down negative emotions makes that energy deplete even faster. If you're caught in the middle of a downward communication spiral with someone—getting angry, making personal attacks, drumming up the past—call a halt and agree on an amount of time that the two of you will take before resuming the issue. This could be anywhere from an hour to a week or more, depending on what feels right. You might choose to spend the time doing something that increases your emotional frequency—exercising, playing video games, reading, throwing a private dance party, etc. The idea is that when you come back to it, you'll be calm, collected, and better able to continue talking without biting the other person's head off.

Practice being able to step away from a heated argument. It's much harder than it seems. When you're angry and annoyed, it's likely that the inner voice of your ego is practically screaming, *You can't back down now! You have to win! You have to make sure he knows that you're right and he's wrong!* That inner voice, left unacknowledged or unchecked, can win a lot of battles while simultaneously losing the connection with the people around you. When the vicious fighter that is your ego is turning up the volume in your head, it's crucial to have some strategies for letting your calm, cool, collected self be the one who does the talking instead.

How to Say It

There are numerous techniques for improving communication, or the *how* part of all of this. You can find plenty of articles, blog posts, books, workshops, and more information about communication hacks in the Resources section. When an uncomfortable or conflict-heavy conversation is headed your way, it's best to have a communication tool (or many tools) to keep you on track and grounded.

Find an established set of tools or a particular communication system to rely on, especially when discussing emotionally intense topics. I prefer to use nonviolent communication (NVC) as a ritual to keep me in line and prevent me from slipping into emotionally driven communication. There is a plethora of resources out there for learning all about this particular technique. NVC stresses the importance of communicating with compassion instead of with combative or violent behavior. There are four primary steps to employing NVC:

First, state an observation of what happened, free of interpretation, accusation, or spin. It's important that the observation be made as objectively as possible, with "I-statements" rather than "you-statements."

"We had plans to go out on a date Tuesday night. Thirty minutes before we were supposed to meet, I received a text from you, canceling."

Second, express your feelings without applying any story about something that was done *to* you by others. This one takes practice. It's very easy to slip into passively accusatory statements such as "I felt abandoned" (translation: "You abandoned me") or "I felt judged" (translation: "You were judging me").

"I felt surprised, lonely, and sad."

"I felt frustrated and disappointed."

Third, express what you need. This is based on what you need to know or feel, rather than how you think your partner needs to behave.

"I need to know that our plans are important enough to you to keep them. I need to feel considered by you."

Lastly, make a request that is not a demand or an ultimatum. Your partner should feel free to either say yes, say no, or negotiate a compromise.

"If you need to reschedule a date of ours, and it's not an emergency, I request you give me at least a day's notice beforehand."

NVC takes practice before it becomes second nature, and it will require you to slow down and be very mindful when you're in the midst of an argument. In my personal experience, NVC can be an excellent tool that allows you to present your perspective in a way that's organized and nonconfrontational, even if your partner hasn't studied it at all. You can find a recap of this and more information at the official website for the Center for Nonviolent Communication at cnvc.org.

Check out the Resources section to find other tools for communication and conflict resolution. You may find that certain techniques work great, and others are just not for you. Employing a technique such as NVC may solve most of your communication problems, or you may find that it drives you nuts. Or you may end up using a blend of many different techniques. The ultimate goal is clarity and compassion:

"Let reciprocity and understanding be your polestar. If a disagreement occurs with you and any of your partners, don't walk away from it until you are absolutely certain that you are both talking about the same thing, and that you both understand where the other person stands on the matter and how important it really is to them. The greatest wounds in ethical relationships come not from true, real breaches of trust, but from miscommunications where a breach of trust is perceived in error. Develop excellent communication with all partners, as early as possible, and cultivate your communication just as carefully as you cultivate your overall rapport.**"** —Mia

---

Twenty-first Century Conflict Resolution

Relationship expert Dr. Pat Allen offers surprising advice for people who get particularly emotional during conflict resolution with their partner. Allen recommends going into separate rooms and taking turns writing long-format messages to each other via email, instant messaging, or text messaging. Conventional wisdom discourages solving conflict in any medium that isn't face-to-face. However, being in separate rooms and communicating only via text gives you physical separation, forces you to slow down and frame your thoughts completely, and eliminates demonstrative displays of negative emotions to your partner, such as raising your voice or aggressive body language. While you may be in separate rooms, you are still able to come together once everything has been talked out to reconnect and clarify anything that may have been lost through text.[1]

Bear in mind that this may not be a go-to technique for every relationship or every disagreement. But if you're finding yourself or your partner bogged down in negative emotion every time you discuss a certain topic, give Dr. Allen's tip a try!

You are the champion of scheduling and planning, but you also know when to be flexible.

Multiple relationships mean a lot of scheduling. The more people involved, the more schedules that need to be taken into consideration. While you may not be able to keep tabs on everything your partners are doing at all times, it is your responsibility to be at least familiar with work schedules or ongoing time commitments. In case you're wondering, yes, this can take up your brain's RAM very quickly.

Successful poly people pride themselves on being champion schedulers. The easiest hack I've found is having a shared Google Calendar. You can quickly see your partner's schedule without a lot of back and forth about when you are both free. Some people choose to have all or some of their partners on a shared calendar.

On the flip side, no one likes being caught in the matrix of an unbendable schedule. You may have finally gotten your weekend perfectly planned out, then word comes in from the front lines that your girlfriend's work schedule has changed and now instead of Tuesday evening for your date, it can only be Friday evening, which you were planning on spending with your boyfriend. These situations happen all the time.

Flexibility is key. In an ideal world, this wouldn't be happening last minute, and you, your girlfriend, and your boyfriend would have the flexibility to understand rearranging date nights without any feelings getting hurt. But regardless of flexibility and timing, sometimes someone ends up at the crappy end of the scheduling stick. If Friday evening is your boyfriend's birthday and you've had surprise plans for him for months, you may have to make the choice to maintain that time commitment instead of moving it around. You may have to wait until next week to see your girlfriend.

These scheduling conflict situations are par for the course in managing multiple relationships. Depending on the circumstances, they can either be like water off a duck's back, or a potential source for anger and frustration for everyone involved. It's hard to give advice that would cover all situations and every factor that could potentially be involved. At the end of the day, choosing flexibility is much more likely to bring happiness and peace to you and your partners. If you are on the receiving end of a scheduling snafu, maintain trust in your partner's love even if your date has to be moved to another day. If you have a partner who is feeling put out by a scheduling mishap, put effort toward reassurance and instilling him or her with confidence in your care.

¡Sí se puede!

No, I'm not saying you have to be bilingual to have great relationships. "Sí se puede" was originally the motto of the United Farm Workers, coined by civil rights activist Cesar Chavez during his twenty-four day fast in 1972. It has been translated many different ways, generally to the tune of "Yes, it is possible," or "Yes, we can."[2] The phrase has its own Wikipedia entry, and this is my favorite part:

> *The saying Sí Se Puede has long been a UFW guiding principle that has served to inspire accomplishment of goals even in what at times may seem insurmountable situations.*[3]

I love that.

For me, saying "Sí se puede" or "Yes, we can" isn't just a verbal pump-up or inspirational mantra. It perfectly embodies a trait known as *self-efficacy*. Self-efficacy is a mix of confidence, self-esteem, and the ability to bounce back from setbacks.

For example, let's say this section of the book inspires you to go take a Spanish class. If you go into your Spanish class with the inherent belief that there is no way you can actually learn the language, knowing you've always been terrible at languages, and that this class is unlikely to be useful or effective, then guess what? You're probably going to come out of that Spanish class having learned very little. *No bueno.* But if you believe that you do have the capability to learn Spanish, even if you have a history of difficulty in language classes, you will learn much more, much faster, and much more effectively. Several studies corroborate this phenomenon.[4]

So where do non-monogamous relationships come into all this? For most people, entering into a poly relationship involves a lot of learning—learning about yourself, learning to manage emotions, learning to communicate better, learning how to love many people without hurting them or yourself. The stakes are a little bit higher than in Spanish class. That's a lot of learning to do, and many people squash their own success before they even try.

"I am way too jealous of a person."

"I can't stand the thought of my partner going on a date with someone else."

"I don't want to know about or meet my partner's other partners. I couldn't handle the awkwardness."

These sentiments are all too common, and I can tell you that most people who have repeatedly expressed variations of the above to me ended up having a disastrous first foray into non-monogamy.

Open relationships require you to extend yourself outside of your comfort zone and to do and feel things that may be completely new and totally foreign. The common thread in great poly relationships, whether the people in them have been doing it for decades or just for a few months, is that confidence in knowing that they have the capability to handle whatever arises. Even if it's totally new. Even if it's awkward and uncomfortable. Even if it's terrifying.

So how do you get self-efficacy in the face of new emotional challenges? Most people establish a strong or weak sense of self-efficacy in childhood and their formative years, but there are still many options for developing it as an adult. You may examine what negative recurring thoughts you have about yourself and choose to keep a positive-thought journal to unknit that neural pathway. Or you may take stock of your accomplishments and strengths and make the effort to remind yourself of what you've overcome whenever you're overwhelmed by the task at hand. (Can you have self-efficacy about learning to have self-efficacy? Like a meta-self-efficacy? Mind=blown.)

You can embrace the emotional equivalent of being buck naked at school in the middle of puberty.

Sorry if that caused any involuntary shudders.

A radically honest relationship format will take every single insecurity you have and drag it out into the spotlight. That probably sounds pretty terrifying, and it is.

Let's say one of my partners starts dating someone new, and I find myself awkward and tense around her, even though she is kind and gregarious to me. Upon first impression, I notice that this new partner is gorgeous, just got her PhD in physics, and has a successful, well-paying career. Immediately the inner peanut gallery starts up:

> *Ugh, I'm ten pounds heavier than I want to be. Why didn't I go after a graduate degree? I'm going to end up on food stamps. Why would my partner want to be with someone as fat, dumb, poor, and lame as me? He's probably going to leave me for her.*

The script writer in your head has a flair for melodrama.

When your inner voice of insecurity is going from zero to sixty, it changes everything if you make the choice to be vulnerable and share it with your partner. Don't internalize it. Don't pout. Don't passively take it out on your partner or on your partner's new paramour. Share it.

And keep in mind, you aren't sharing these things with your partner hoping that the result will be that he cancels the hot date lined up for tonight, or ends a new relationship. When you share the icky, self-conscious bits of your being with someone you love, it gives both of you the opportunity to collaborate on ways to help both of you feel secure and supported, without needing to break any hearts.

This could be as simple as verbal reassurance from your partner that you are loved, that you should be proud of your accomplishments, or that he or she finds you incredibly sexy, especially when you smile. It could be making the decision to connect more with your partner's new partner to help quell some of those fears surrounding this new person. (More on meeting metamours in chapter 10.) Or it might lay the groundwork for your partner to share some similar fears and insecurities with you.

Vulnerability is uncomfortable, but it doesn't have to be feared. If anything, it should be embraced as an opportunity to get closer to your partners and to begin shaping new thought patterns around your insecurities.

You are willing to continually build your empathy and compassion muscles.

The reasons to be compassionate to others could take up a whole other book. That topic alone is the basis for many religious texts. From kindergarten we all get the same message: Play nice. Share. Don't hit your sister. But as adults, those priorities get a little skewed. If you grew up in a highly competitive culture, compassion and empathy are often sacrificed in favor of making sure you take care of number one. The message is different: Get to the top. Get that promotion. Protect what's yours. Don't let anyone take advantage of you.

Don't think that those messages are only present in the aggressive corporate world. Look at how many books and articles are out there about how to land a husband, how to get your boyfriend to settle down, how to make your relationship "affair-proof." Look at how many relationships dissolve into conflict over perceived threats from a flirtatious coworker or from one person reconnecting with an ex-girlfriend. Kindergarten lessons don't hold up in the world of possessive love. The consensus: *compassion and empathy are great for making friends, but you want me to play nice with the bitch who is trying to steal away my partner?!*

Some of the best advice I've ever gotten came from Franklin Veaux, author of several books on polyamory and the polyamory advice website *More Than Two.* Veaux said, "Reach for the most compassionate version of yourself. You're doing this because you love people."[5] There will be times when you don't get exactly what you want. There will be times when you feel like someone else is getting something that you don't have—sex, affection, quality time. There will be times when you feel like things are unfair—your partner has an awesome first date, and you get stood up. In these times, it's so important to step away from the standard narrative of taking all you can and looking out for number one in order to draw on your reserves of compassion.

Many people insist that non-monogamy is inherently full of conflict and negativity. Surely someone's feelings are bound to get hurt. In any relationship feelings do get hurt and mistakes are made, but there is no universal law dictating that adding more people to the picture means adding more quarrels and pain.

One of the primary distinguishing points that separates ethical non-monogamy from traditional relationships is a sense that you, your partners, and your partners' partners are all on the same team. In an ideal world, you are all striving for the same goal—happiness, peace, and abundance for everyone. It requires choosing cohesion over conflict, choosing connection over competition. It requires seeking to understand the feelings of others, and the courage to be generous and loving even when you don't feel like it. This may sound corny, but there really isn't any other way for human beings to successfully coexist, within relationships or otherwise.

Be clear on your personal boundaries. Don't be a doormat. Never allow yourself to be abused. But when you're in a tense situation, feeling jealous or insecure, or upset over a perceived fault, consider choosing warmth, compassion, and empathy over the alternative.

"*Don't think of yourself first too much. You are in teams now and you have to act like a player with team spirit, although you should also communicate your limits and what is of prime importance to you.***"**—Bea

The Just Be Nice Campaign

Meditation and mindfulness teacher Jessica Graham created a technique for generating compassion in her own relationships:

"*I was feeling really focused on what I didn't like about my relationship. I didn't want it to end, but I didn't feel great in it either. I tried something that I***

have actually suggested to others for years. It's the "Just Be Nice" campaign. It's just what it sounds like. I was just nice. When I got annoyed, scared, frustrated, felt not heard, got triggered—I was just nice. Sometimes that meant leaving the room for a moment, but no matter what I was just nice. I focused on being the best partner I could be and took any focus off of what I thought [my partner] was doing wrong. I kept my side of the street clean.

I decided to do this for ninety days. I had a few slip ups but for the most part I did pretty well. I realized that many times it was not necessary to have a big talk about how I was feeling. I still spoke to someone and/or wrote about my feelings, but I didn't take problems or negativity to my partner. I also got more clarity on what was actually a problem and not just me being reactive. At the end of the three months I felt better and my relationship was better.[6]

You've got guts.

Chutzpah. Guts. Nerve. Grit. Audacity. Courage.

Historically, people who go against the grain do not have an easy time of it. Though some would argue that non-monogamy is a more natural behavior for human beings, the majority of Western cultures currently embrace the long-term, monogamous dyad as the hallmark of normalcy. Straying beyond the bounds of "normal" almost always guarantees reactions ranging from excited, curious fascination to confusion, disgust, and ridicule.

When you are in an alternative relationship, nearly everyone you encounter will have an opinion about it, and sometimes it will be negative. That's where the courage comes in—not to righteously defend yourself or to rip apart that close-minded nitwit criticizing the way you love, but instead to be gracious, kind, and to keep doing you. It's the courage to keep being happy even when someone else says you shouldn't be. The happiest poly people I know take these reactions—the good, the bad, and the ugly—in stride.

Negative reactions can come from other non-monogamous folk too! Even within the poly community, you'll find plenty of people convinced that they have figured out the one right way to do it, and your open relationship may not meet their standards. But the most fulfilled poly relationships are those that are being uniquely created by the people involved to achieve maximum possible happiness for everyone, whatever that may look like. Having the guts to unapologetically create something new (which may take several different experiments) is paramount. There'll be more about building up that gutsy confidence to handle the reactions of others in chapter 9.

Beyond weathering the storm of negative reactions, it takes guts to try something totally new and foreign, such as a radically different approach to relationships after a lifetime of traditional monogamy. It takes *major* guts to face your deep fears surrounding rejection, loss, and personal insecurities. It takes even more guts to let someone you love be free, trusting that they'll still care for you; to leap off the cliff and trust that your wings will sprout on the way down. Throwing your body, heart, and mind into the unknown offers no guarantees, but once you've made it to the other side, the resulting strength and confidence does not easily slip away.

In an acting class years ago, I got an excellent gem of wisdom. At the time it was meant to encourage more risk-taking and making bolder choices in a scene, but I found it to be an excellent piece of life advice: *Whatever it is you are scared to do, that is the thing that you must do next.*

You're excited to date yourself.

First dates. Some people love them, some people hate them. Personally, I get a lot of enjoyment out of the process of just getting to know someone. Beyond discovering surface-level similarities between myself and my date such as favorite movies, musical preferences, or a shared love of Vietnamese food, I love asking my date questions about their upbringing, about the craziest, wildest hopes they have for their life, their deepest or weirdest fears, and their philosophies surrounding spirituality or self-development.

When we start falling in love with someone, every unique facet that we encounter can become interesting and endearing—their secret obsession with Taylor Swift music, their dedication to daily meditation, or the way they talk to their three dogs. These are the puzzle pieces that put together a human being, from deep foundational beliefs to silly idiosyncrasies and habits. It's the sum of these parts in someone else that we fall in love with.

You, too, are made up of all these puzzle pieces. And it's just as important to become familiar with your own ins and outs as it is when getting to know a potential mate. You may be incredulous. After all, you've been stuck with yourself your entire life, and you just slogged through all of the self-inquiry questions in chapter 3. Surely you're pretty well acquainted with yourself by now!

The things that make you *you* are constantly shifting and changing. The version of you from ten years ago, the person you were when you ended your last relationship, and the you who woke up this morning probably all have very different romantic and sexual needs, different strengths and weaknesses, different preferences and philosophies about life and love. Getting to know yourself is an endless, and endlessly fascinating, lifelong journey.

So keep up that curiosity about yourself, the same way you are curious to learn about a lover. If you've never been excited by the idea of getting flowers from your partner, but your knees turn to custard every time he compliments the way you look, take note and investigate! (Hint: It might have something to do with your love language. Or an extreme pollen allergy.) If you get turned on by getting to hear about your partner's sexual attraction to other people, but get paralyzed with jealousy or fear if you find out the person your partner is dating has a much higher income than you, take some time to look inward. If, upon examination, you realize that you've had a long-standing insecurity surrounding money and self-worth, that gives you access to not only start undoing the negative thought pattern but also open up to your partner about it. Instead of being a slave to the emotional trigger, you have an in to fixing it, adjusting it, or re-directing it. This is a priceless resource when you're in the process of turning jealousy around—something covered extensively in chapter 5.

"Dating yourself" goes beyond getting to know yourself; it also means taking care of yourself. Self-care practices look different depending on what your personal needs are, but generally you should strive to give your body what it needs to be healthy, your mind what it needs to be peaceful and focused, and your soul what it needs to feel content. If you are hurting in any of these arenas, it will be doubly difficult to care for others in your life. A large part of my personal self-care involves having alone time. When I don't actually schedule "me time," it quickly fills up with obligations to partners, projects, friends, and others, and I find myself depleted.

Self-care Commitment Challenge

Historically, men have been expected to act as breadwinners and women have been expected to act as caregivers, dedicating their time and energy to their spouse, children, aging parents, and other family members. Living under this expectation has led many women to neglect self-care or to feel that doing something for themselves is selfish.

Even if you don't consciously feel any guilt about taking time for yourself, it's easy to let obligations to work, family, friends, partners, and other commitments fill up the schedule, leaving no room for "me time." As you add more romantic partners to your life, it can become even more difficult to carve out time for self-care.

If you want to take time for yourself but have no idea where to start, try out the Self-care Commitment Challenge:

1. Set aside a thirty-minute block of time each day to dedicate to self-care. I'd recommend waking up half an hour earlier and making it part of your morning routine. If the morning is not feasible, find a time that you can set consistently for each day.
2. Pick one to three activities to do during this half-hour window that make you feel joyful, peaceful, fulfilled, relaxed, or generally positive. For a long time, my morning self-care routine involved ten minutes of meditation, ten minutes of free writing, and ten minutes of sun salutations. You may choose to spend the whole thirty minutes reading poetry, going for a walk by yourself, or even masturbating!
3. Do your self-care routine for thirty days. At the end of thirty days, evaluate what worked and what didn't. You may change the time of day or the self-care activities depending on what's most effective for you.

You have a little bit of Zen.

Disclaimer: For many years I've identified as "Buddh-ish." I am wary of unquestioningly subscribing to every piece of dogma touted by any religious institution, but my spiritual streak is still strong. I'm a longtime practitioner of meditation, and the tenets of Buddhism closely align with my own ideals . . . just not perfectly enough to make me a devout convert. So don't take this section as some kind of missionary work for a particular religious practice or a request to put your faith in a deity. That's a journey for you to take on your own.

Zen (or enlightenment, inner peace, balance, being strong in the Force, or whatever you want to call it) is the through-line that glues together all of the skills and qualities listed above. Zen is traditionally difficult to define. Some have called it "divine confusion." There's a long-running practice of Zen masters delivering impenetrable koans or riddles to their students, which force them into enlightenment through the sheer perplexity that comes from trying to pin down the what, where, how, and why of Zen. To step out of the philosophical realm of the guru pretzeled up on the yoga mat and into the practical world of negotiating relationships, having a little bit of Zen boils down to three practices: equanimity, conscious awareness, and staying present.

Equanimity is the state in which you are able to enjoy the good parts of life without desperately clinging to them, and to weather the bad parts without kicking and screaming. It's what enables you to bask in the delicious glow that is your partner's love without feeling the need to keep her under your thumb to make sure she'll never leave you. It's what gets you through a night of loneliness after your date canceled on you and all of your partners are off with someone else. It's what allows you to brush off hurtful or judgmental comments made by those skeptical of your relationship choices. Equanimity can be found from a wide variety of access points—developing a personal spiritual practice, creating affirmations, connecting with a solid support network, reading philosophy, educating yourself on positive psychology, and many others.

Conscious awareness encompasses the awareness you have of yourself as well as others around you. It drives the ability to objectively watch negative emotional reactions such as jealousy or anxiety without acting on them or taking them out on your partner. It lets you soak in the positive feelings that come after a night of wonderful sex for the first time with a new partner, or to more acutely enjoy the warmth you feel when coming home to your partner of ten years. Awareness keeps you in tune with your partners and your metamours, enabling you to be considerate of others' feelings and savvy about small conflicts that need to be solved early in order to prevent bigger conflicts down the road.

Lastly, *staying present* is both extraordinarily important and extraordinarily difficult. The human brain is wired to analyze the past and worry about the future, and this easily infects relationships. Experiencing a relationship in the now, without influence from the past or the future, is nearly impossible. We nurse wounds from ex-boyfriends for years; we fantasize about the wonderful future we might build when a new partner comes along, but also get crushed with anxiety over the notion that our partner may abandon us or not fulfill all of our wishes. We've all mentally carved out ideal versions of the future and how we want our partners to fit into those visions. Many of us have committed the transgression of eagerly awaiting the improved future version of a boyfriend or girlfriend—how great things will be once he gets in shape, or once she gets a job. How many times have you turned down a potential romantic partner because he or she didn't hit every checklist item of what you think a partner should have in order to fit into your future?

If you truly want extraordinary relationships—relationships that are completely of your own making, that defy the odds, and that wake you up, light you up, and turn you on—you have to start from the present, and only the present. Let go of tightly held baggage from past relationships that is preventing you from opening up your current relationships. Don't let your partner's past mistakes have a lasting hold on your heart, and make a commitment to not dredge up past faults to use as ammo in arguments. Let your future be open, blank, and ripe for every possibility, free from constraints of the past or anxiety over what happens next.

Chapter 4 Homework

Exercise #1

Take some time to mindfully set some commitments or intentions for personal growth. Imagine the best possible version of yourself, and examine what steps will need to be accomplished in order to get there. This visualization can really help shape the kind of commitments you want to make to yourself.

Exercise #2

Think of something that you are afraid of doing. It could be applying for a new job, asking someone out, or sitting at home alone while your partner is out on a date. What limiting beliefs about yourself are holding you back from doing it? (E.g. *I'm not qualified enough. I'm not worthy enough to avoid rejection.*) What would it feel like if you had everything you needed internally in order to face this scary situation head-on? What would happen if you went ahead and did what you're afraid of doing, even before you have all the personal strength you need?

Section III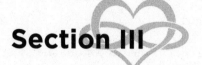

Mastering Non-Monogamy

5 The Biggest Question: Jealousy

"Don't you get jealous?" is the most frequent question someone in a non-monogamous relationship gets asked, hands down. For many people, even thinking about their partner gallivanting with someone else is enough to trigger a gut-wrenching jealous response. And why wouldn't it? In pop culture, there are few widely known examples of non-monogamy turning out to be a *good* thing for everyone involved. Instead, we are exposed to the horror stories—politicians resigning in shame over being caught in an affair, television dramas and big-budget films whose plots revolve entirely around a tumultuous love triangle, distraught married men committing suicide after being exposed by the Ashley Madison hack, and innumerable personal tales of deception, infidelity, and heartbreak.

These painful experiences are characterized not just by jealousy, but by the tangled mix of agonizing feelings that are intertwined with jealousy—feeling betrayed, abandoned, crushed from losing a partner, embarrassed over being fooled, and ashamed of not being enough. Contrary to popular belief, even people who have been in polyamorous relationships for decades still experience jealousy. However, you will find in this chapter that jealousy is intricate, comprising many moving parts and slippery emotions. In learning to deconstruct the parts of jealousy, you also will learn how to tackle the little (or big) mental quirks and hang-ups that feed it.

Women and Jealousy

All human beings experience jealousy in some form and with different levels of intensity, but women in particular have gotten a bad rap. Everyone is familiar with the trope of the "catty" woman. The term "catty" is only ever applied to women, and the specific cat-like qualities the term conjures up are not exactly flattering—sweet, cuddly, and charming in one moment, but a snarling, yowling, hissing bundle of claws and teeth in the next.

This two-faced duality is present in many stereotypes about women. Think of how frequently women are associated with being emotional, prone to mood swings, and making the people around them wary of their mercurial hormones. It's embodied in the very concept of a "frenemy"—when you're friendly to a person's face while still harboring a sense of rivalry or bitterness toward them.

Jealousy is one of the outstanding characteristics of the catty woman. She keeps an eye on her man at all times, suspicious of any contact with ex-girl-friends and distrustful of his female coworkers. She also gets jealous of what other women have—great looks, a good job, attention from others, or the right wardrobe—and will make passive-aggressive remarks or gossip to others about it. All other women are a potential threat either to her own sense of self or to her relationship.

It makes me cringe, but this is a pretty accurate description of the person that I used to be. I grew up in a household of all women, and made friends eas-ily with other girls when I was growing up. But as many girls find, it became a whole different game in high school. Other girls became competitors in a fierce and unending rivalry for attention, particularly from boys. You must strive to stand out by having the best makeup, flawless skin, the most flattering clothes, and an appealing body. And every fashion magazine was happy to help by offering hundreds of tips on how to tease him, please him, and how to look *perfect* while doing it.

By the time I reached college, I considered jealousy a normal and predict-able part of my emotional makeup. I harbored resentment toward my boy-friend's exes and stiffened around his female friends who, to me, were getting a little *too* friendly. I hated the thought of my boyfriend looking at porn, because I knew that there was no way my body could ever seem as pleasurable or allur-ing as a porn star's. I didn't just compare my looks to the extremes of porn, but against every other woman I met. I felt good about myself when I came out on top in these comparisons—when I was thinner, or had a prettier face. And I felt uncomfortable when the other side was superior—when she was taller, or had thinner legs, or larger breasts. My insecurities and lack of confidence in myself dictated the extent to which I would get jealous, which would then dic-tate how I treated the other person, whether that was my boyfriend, his female friends, a female coworker, or whoever.

The troubling thing is that this behavior was encouraged. The women around me joined me in chiding any man who kept in touch with his ex and shaming women who tried to maintain friendships with guys who were "taken." It was perfectly reasonable to see a well-dressed, put-together, flirtatious woman and label her as "slutty." Like many people, my insecurities and jealousy, fueled by a culture of competition and excessive beauty standards, fostered an environment where it was okay for me to act out, berate my boyfriend for being attracted to other people, and judge other women, which in turn continued to fuel that same negative culture.

Jealousy as Love

While jealousy was an everyday occurrence for me, I was constantly baffled by the lack of jealousy in whoever my boyfriend was at the time. At least on the outside, these guys were as cool as a cucumber! I could talk about other men I found attractive, surround myself with male friends who were clearly interested in being more than friends, and even make out with other guys on stage or in acting class. Wouldn't bat an eye. At the time, this sent me into an even deeper spiral of insecurity and self-doubt. If he's not jealous, that means he doesn't care what I do, that means he's not invested in the relationship, that means *he doesn't really love me.*

It's alarming how frequently jealousy is misconstrued as love. No one wants to have a hyper-jealous, possessive, and controlling partner, but there's a general agreement that if your partner really cares about you and doesn't want to lose you, there should be at least some displays of jealousy. If strangers at the bar start checking you out or if your coworker is getting flirty, it's expected that there should *at least* be a passive comment, maybe a puffing out of the chest and setting of the jaw. I can't even recall the number of times I've heard a friend say something along the lines of "I told my boyfriend about the guy who asked for my number, and he got jealous! It was so cute!"

Much of this stems from archaic notions of romantic male chivalry. The knight swoops in to defend his maiden from bandits, dragons, and (most importantly) the other horny knights.

The romance of a man guarding his treasured damsel is a well-spun thread, but the idea of a woman guarding her partner holds much of the same allure. The story is appealing—you protect the person you love from any threats, real or imagined. It shows how much you are willing to fight for them and how much you must really love them.

This positive, romantic spin on jealousy feeds a culture of justification for bad behavior. The guy who admonishes his girlfriend for wearing a short dress is just trying to protect her from other men who would take advantage of her. The wife who stalks her husband's female friends on social media is only doing it because of how much she doesn't want to lose him. Jealousy can bring out the worst in us—the person inside that's afraid, trapped, insecure, and will stop at nothing to feel safe again. But we hold up our love for the other person, our concern, our noble side, to mask the small, scared, jealous person inside. "I only get jealous because of how much I love you!" At the end of the day, who could argue with such a supposedly loving person?

Where Does Jealousy Come From?

To function in a non-monogamous relationship, it is necessary to strip away this facade of nobility. Jealousy may bring out one's icky parts, but it doesn't mean that it's something to be ashamed of. It is an emotion that is perfectly natural for all human beings to feel at some point—the same way that all human beings are capable of feeling sadness, anger, fear, disgust, ecstasy, and excitement.

It is, however, a fundamentally complex emotion. The term "jealousy" itself gives us a clue as to the circumstances surrounding the emotion. The various dictionary definitions of the word have a common through-line: someone else has something that you want, or is threatening to take away something that you have. But the term itself doesn't reveal what's actually going on below the surface. There are many inroads to jealousy, and every individual can be triggered by totally unique circumstances that may link back to childhood memories, trauma from past relationships, or any number of strange quirks embedded in one's emotional makeup. However, the most common hang-ups that trigger jealousy are comparisons, competition, fear, and loss of control.

Comparison and What It Means

Have you ever wondered how you would feel about different aspects of yourself— your body, your house, your job, your fashion sense, your bank account—if there were no one else around to compare them to? Would you even know if you were poor or rich? If you were overweight, fit, or skinny? If your actions were right or wrong?

It's mind-boggling to imagine not having anyone else around for comparison, because comparison is an intrinsic mental process that enables us to define ourselves and our place in the world. We evaluate nearly every aspect of ourselves based on the context and the people that surround us.[1] Comparison is rudimentary observation: *This person is older than me. That person has darker skin than me. That person is driving an Audi, and I am not.* But the next step is to apply *meaning* to the comparison, which is where it gets tricky.

You might make a simple comparison between yourself and someone your partner is dating, such as:

This person has longer and wavier hair than I do.

Which then has meaning applied to it and gets turned into this:

This person has longer and wavier hair than I do . . . her hair looks so much healthier than mine. She looks way better in pictures than I do. She's so much more attractive than me. My boyfriend is going to find her prettier than me, and he's going to give her more attention, and like her more, and eventually break up with boring ol' me.

And thus we've gone from looking at someone and noticing that their hair is different to wallowing in dread over the day your boyfriend leaves you for Miss Shampoo Commercial.

Social media is prime territory for this. The majority of us are masterful at tailoring a picture-perfect online presence. We post the pictures where we look the most attractive, like we're having the most fun, have the best friends, and generally have the most rewarding, exciting life anyone could ask for. If anyone is going to compare themselves to the online version of ourselves, we want to come out ahead. And we use it to fuel the inner comparison-making engine all the time—checking up on exes and scoping out the girl who keeps liking all of your boyfriend's pictures.

Online and offline, comparisons are unavoidable. There are billions of other human beings out there, and surprise surprise, they're all a little bit different from you. Some people will be prettier, richer, or more successful than you, and others will not be as healthy, as smart, or as good at karaoke as you are. However, the *meaning* that you apply to these comparisons is what makes the difference between feeling good about yourself and falling into a death spiral of jealousy and insecurity.

Having high self-esteem is useful for maintaining positivity and avoiding the temptation to negatively compare yourself to others, but it isn't a cure-all by itself. I've felt absolutely great about my body . . . until I saw that my meta-mour had better-defined abs. By all means, embrace yourself, love yourself, and find your strengths in order to boost your confidence, but be aware that *genuine* self-esteem is something that is still there even when everyone around you seems to be making you look bad.

Why make all these comparisons? Why is it so easy to squirm at the thought of your partner dating someone who looks like a supermodel? Besides the meanings we apply to our everyday comparisons, we also apply the stakes that come from competition.

High-stakes Competition

Sociologists and psychologists cite the social theory of comparison—the theory that we constantly compare ourselves to other human beings to determine our status, rank, or place in the world, so that we may then increase it.[2] Why increase your rank or better yourself? Because of competition. There's been much research on the ways that animals naturally compete for water, food, mates, shelter, and other resources. Humans have taken competition to the extreme—you can look at the rapidly growing list of species that have gone extinct directly because of how voracious we are in the competition for land and natural resources. Much of this is fueled by scarcity, both real and imagined. If you think there isn't enough to go around, you have to make sure to get yours.

This attitude of scarcity is often applied to love, sex, affection, and com-panionship. There's a feeling of lack that is sprinkled into our romantic rela-tionships. You need to claim your portion of love before someone else gets it. You need find the person who will emotionally take care of you, love you, cuddle you, sexually satisfy you, help raise your children, and have your back, because no one else will. This is why the very thought of polyamory is threat-ening to many people. It's difficult enough to secure a reliable lover in this world . . . how could you let someone else tap into *your* source of love, sex, and affection? The well will run dry!

If you believe that love is hard to come by, it is quite natural to become possessive. Like a toddler clutching a toy, we cling to people and relationships, shouting at the rest of the world, "This is mine! Back off! Go get your own!" It is wrapped up in the way we talk about love; think about how many love songs mention wanting to make him or her "mine." And forget about having to "share" your partner with someone else. We all remember what a bummer it was in preschool when the teacher asked you to share your toys. For many people, the extent of one's love directly correlates to how tightly one can hold on to the object of their affection.

The problem is that people are not property, and love is not a limited resource. People can't really be given, taken, stolen like treasure, won like a prize, or shared like a toy. The capacity to give and receive love is infinite and abundant. You came into this world with the ability to love and be loved by a wide circle of friends, each newly born family member, and multiple lovers and partners, both simultaneously and over the course of your entire life.

So why do we still think about love as every woman for herself? What makes us look at other people as competitors in a never-ending contest for love and attention?

Fear

Our impulses to compare and compete are driven by our fears. Yes, it's a no-brainer, and we are all familiar with the ubiquitous message of every motivational speaker: *Fear not! Feel the fear and do it anyway! The only thing we have to fear is fear itself!* So much easier said than done.

Jealousy arises out of fears that are usually well-established in one's psychological makeup from an early age. This can be a deep-rooted fear of abandonment, implanted by the death or departure of a parent. It can be triggered by fears of being replaced by a newer model (who might literally look like a model), or fears of your partner not finding you special or unique. Jealousy can come from fears of being left out and left behind, being stuck at home with the dirty dishes while your partner is off having all the fun with a hot date. Or you may be afraid that you can't trust your partner as far as you can throw him. If you've been betrayed, lied to, cheated on in the past, it is all too easy to assume that the same nightmare will happen again.

When we get jealous and feel afraid of losing the love-competition to others, of being seen unfavorably in a comparison, or that we're going to be left utterly alone, every muscle and fiber in the body gets ready to take action. When caught in the throes of jealousy, the body produces the classic fight-or-flight response that happens whenever we're afraid. However, the endocrine system does not differentiate between different fearful scenarios, and it releases immunity-compromising stress hormones whether we are experiencing "true" fear (fear that arises in actual life-threatening situations such as a car accident, being physically assaulted, falling, etc.) or "false" fear (fear that arises when you have to give a presentation at work, when you're asking someone out on a date, or when you worry that your partner will leave you for someone else). Our fears, big or small, not only leave us vulnerable to disease, but can hobble our ability to have healthy, trustworthy, stable relationships.

Giving Permission to Break Your Heart

Our jealousies are nearly always linked to our deeply held fears. Dr. Lissa Rankin, author of *The Fear Cure*, discusses the ways in which our fears can poison our relationships, as well as compromise our mental and physical health. Dr. Rankin proposes allowing our fears to teach us exactly what it is we need to address within ourselves in order to remove our barriers to happiness. Heartbreak and loss crack us open, and in that crack we can witness who we really are, what we really need, and find so many more opportunities to continue to live and love, even when we feel like shutting everything out. She even proposes granting permission to break your heart—to a pet, to a child, to a new romantic partner.[3] When you give your permission to let someone break your heart, you willingly accept that even though there may be pain in the future, it is something to be embraced and used for growth and understanding, not something to fear.

Loss of Control and Regaining Control

The comparisons, competition, and fears that make up our jealousy response act as a glaring highlight of the lack of control that we have within relationships. Your partner may very well dump you, or she may fall head over heels for her athletic and charismatic personal trainer, or may one day decide that she's bored with living with you and wants to move across the country. The deep, uncomfortable truth that we all know but never want to acknowledge is that *there is nothing you can do to prevent it.*

Anyone who enters a relationship with you is their own person, with their own needs and desires, quirks and hang-ups, and with a completely unique and unpredictable life path to follow. You can't make your partner love you any more or less, and you can't make your partner love anyone else more or

less. Factor in the inability to foresee drastic curves in the road such as illness, job opportunities, or death, and you're looking at a slippery, unknown
future in any relationship. Until the day it's possible to order up a perfect robot
love-slave, programmed to give you everything you need with no wants of its
own, we're all looking at a future where no relationship is objectively stable,
unchanging, or permanent. (Even then, the robot love-slave is bound to break
down now and then.) Ultimately, you have no control whatsoever over your
partner and your partner's decisions. Change, for better or worse, is inevitable.

A truth like that does not sit well with anybody. Fear, jealousy, and loss
of control are unpleasant, nauseating feelings. It's no surprise that when these
feelings bubble up, priority number one is to make it stop, *now*. In our desperate attempts to quell these uncomfortable emotions, we tend to shoot first, ask
questions later.

Solutions to Jealousy (That Don't Solve Anything)

The discomfort of jealousy can be as small as a quick twinge in your chest, or as
big as being broadsided by a wave of panicked sickness and endless knots in your
stomach. Either way, not a lot of fun. There are a number of solutions that many
people turn to in order to quell these feelings as fast as possible. In reality, these
solutions are akin to slapping a Band-Aid on a patient suffering from internal
bleeding. They have the appearance of being a fix without addressing the actual
underlying issue. In scrambling to regain emotional balance and get back in control, it is common to grasp at whatever's around to pull you back up again. This
can lead to short-sighted rules, restrictions, knee-jerk reactions, and other inflexible relationship structures. These are covered in detail in chapter 7, but most of
them fall into three general categories: controlling information, controlling your
partner, or controlling the relationship.

Controlling Information

Sometimes information is the target of our desperate grasps at control. If the
knowledge that your partner is rolling around in bed with a hot new lover has
your throat tight and your stomach turning, it is all too logical to conclude that
it would be better if you just didn't have to know. This is usually the basis for
creating Don't Ask, Don't Tell rules (see chapter 7). Requiring your partner to
cover any evidence of being with someone else is the hallmark of denial. I have

yet to meet someone who insisted on not knowing any information about their partner's other relationships who was also quite happy and content with being non-monogamous.

On the other end of the spectrum, some people seek to regain control by requiring that they get information about everything. This can manifest as needing to hear every detail of the sex your partner had with someone else, requiring that you get to read every text exchange your partner has with another, obsessively stalking metamours on social media, or even resorting to snooping through your partner's phone or email in order to get the full story.

The tell-me-every-last-little-thing approach can be motivated by a variety of reasons. If you're like me, you feel that if you know something ahead of time, you can be prepared for it. Knowing everything means no surprises, no getting caught off guard, and not having to be vulnerable. Or you may construe your partner's privacy and autonomy within other relationships as being secretive, untrustworthy, or a method to keep information from you.

Unfortunately, neither of these tactics actually solves the causes of jealousy, and often they create more problems. Asking your partner to protect your feelings by excluding all information forces him to lie to you, omit details, and cripple his ability to be totally open and honest with you. Asking for too much information violates the autonomy and independence of your partner and his other partners. When entering a relationship, you expect a certain level of privacy—that your boyfriend won't reveal personal information or show steamy sexting exchanges to his buddies or family members. The same rings true here. If you have established a relationship wherein you and your partner share absolutely everything with each other, either reconsider that agreement or make sure that you inform all of your other partners of this fact. Although don't expect many people to be comfortable knowing that their private conversations with you are always privy to a third party. And of course, snooping through your partner's stuff in the pursuit of information is the ultimate invasion of privacy.

Snooping

As our personal lives and social interactions migrate into the digital realm, the temptation to snoop through a partner's email, text messages, or social media accounts is greater than ever before. One study in the UK found that 34 percent of women and 62 percent of men had snooped on a partner at one point.[4] Most people are motivated by trying to find out if their partner is cheating on them. If you're in a non-monogamous relationship where nothing is being hidden, that eliminates the primary incentive for snooping. Despite this, some people still choose to invade their partner's privacy to keep tabs on what's going on in other relationships.

If you find yourself tempted to snoop through your partner's personal information or private conversations, take time to stop and ask yourself a few questions to get to the bottom of your temptation. Is it because you're feeling jealous or insecure? What do you expect to find? What are you desperately hoping you won't find? Is it just out of curiosity? Is it motivated by your partner acting suspiciously? The answers to these questions will act as a starting point for having an open conversation with your partner about your feelings and desire to snoop. If there is specific suspicious behavior from your partner prompting your feelings, consult the section in chapter 4 on nonviolent communication to learn how to present your observations in a non-threatening way.

If you are concerned about your partner snooping on you, remember this old proverb: *Don't tie your shoes in a watermelon field.* You may not spend much time in watermelon fields these days, so I'll explain. A person who stops to tie his shoes in a watermelon field looks exactly the same as a person who is bending down to steal a watermelon. Even though tying your shoes is an innocent act, there's still a risk of the watermelon farmer sending the dogs after you to chase you down. Even if you have nothing to hide from your partner, you may be unintentionally giving shady vibes. When you are communicating remotely with another partner, it helps to over-communicate. It can be as simple as "Hey, Aaron just texted me. Give me a sec to respond," or "Lara is asking me about what time would be best for me to pick her up on Saturday." There should not be a need to show entire conversations to your partner, but honestly sharing about your relationships and digital communications will foster trust.

Controlling Your Partner

Instead of seeking to control information, many people try to directly or indirectly control their partner. So many restrictive rules are laid down in relationships for this very reason. The idea of letting your partner pursue whoever they want is frightening, so rules are set in place that dictate not only who your partner can date, but also how they can interact with them. This can include requiring that your partner ask your permission before going out with someone; running any potential partners by you for approval first; requiring them to avoid particular activities with other partners such as spending the night, certain sex positions, or using pet names; or forbidding them from falling in love with anyone else.

A more indirect way of controlling your partner is by choosing to make her wrong. This means projecting your negative feelings, leveling shame, guilt, or personal attacks, and blaming your partner for making you feel jealous. The thinking is, "I feel hurt, therefore she hurt me," or "I feel jealous and insecure, therefore she made me feel jealous and insecure." At best, this results in your partner getting defensive and walking on eggshells, unable to feel free to act for fear of upsetting you. At worst, this results in your partner going underground and finding more creative ways to conceal any information that would result in a blowup.

Controlling the Relationship

Lastly, many people seek to control their jealousy by controlling the entire shape and function of the relationship itself. Some choose monogamy purely because of their fear of experiencing jealousy and insecurity. Some people even choose to share a home, get married, or have kids with someone for the purpose of securing the relationship and preventing feelings of jealousy. However, there are many people out there in monogamous relationships who would attest that monogamy is certainly not a perfect cure for uncomfortable feelings.

Some people try to prevent jealousy by forcing the shape of a relationship to be completely fair and equal. As in, you can only go out on a date on Friday if I have a date of my own lined up for Friday as well. If my date cancels on me, you need to cancel on your date. You can only spend the night elsewhere if I have someone else to spend the night with too. This rigid egalitarianism can also extend to multiple partners: everyone gets two nights a week, no more, no less. The same amount of money, time, and effort is doled out to every partner. This desire to balance the scales is explored more in chapter 8.

For couples who are opening up a previously closed relationship, controlling the relationship usually means creating a new relationship structure that will assure that the central relationship remains the most important. This can take the form of restrictive rules or exclusionary agreements, such as giving each partner the power to veto any potential new partner, or establishing a strict hierarchy that dictates that the central relationship will be "primary" and all other relationships must give way to the needs and demands of one's primary partner.

These hierarchal arrangements are very easy to cling to, primarily because of the draw of "couple status." The extreme importance of being part of a couple has been spoon-fed to us from day one. The long-term, monogamous, married couple has been held up as the bedrock of society, as the purest and most admirable form of love to aspire to. Not only are we trained to desire couple status, but we ascribe privilege and preference to people who identify as part of a couple. More on hierarchy and couple privilege in chapters 7 and 8.

Non-monogamous people are often asked, "What if your partner falls in love with someone else and leaves you for that person?" The reality is that this scenario, heartbreaking as it is, can happen at any time and within any kind of relationship. There is nothing that can create a magical force field that will keep your partner faithful and constant regardless of the circumstances. Even if you choose to get married. Even if you choose monogamy. Even if you're keeping everything fair and equal. Even if you decide that your relationship is primary.

An Interlude on Nihilism

All this talk about having no power to prevent your partner from leaving you is a bummer. As you start letting go of attachments and thinking more expansively about the nature of romantic relationships, it can be easy to fall into the trap of nihilism. "Everyone I love is either going to leave me or die someday. What's the point in getting attached to anyone or anything?" This line of thought leads some people to withdraw completely, or to become Buddhist monastics, or to keep all relationships at arm's length. But this book is not for those people.

Letting go of control, accepting that you cannot own another person, and realizing that the future will always be uncertain is not the precursor to depression, but a step on the path to emotional liberation. When you are no longer plagued with worry over the future of your relationships, you are able to enjoy them as they are right in this very moment. Make plans, act with intention, and take care of other people's hearts, but let your partners be free, let the future unfold on its own, and keep your love in the present.

Jealousy's Call to Action

Imagine you are looking into a petri dish under a microscope. In the dish are dozens of little single-celled amoebae, swimming and darting about. If you place a drop of sugar water into the dish, the amoebae will flock to it and eagerly start sucking it up. *Yum yum yum yum yum!* If you place a drop of vinegar into the dish, the amoebae will recoil and flee. *Ick ick ick ick ick!*

After millennia of evolution and adaptation (and acquiring a few more cells along the way), human beings still act the same exact way as amoebae do. We spend our lives chasing good feelings, desiring comfort, fun, and pleasure. And we shrink from the nasty feelings, from physical pain and emotional turmoil, from awkward conversations and bitter breakups. In considering polyamory, there is much to be gained: an abundance of love, affection, and attention. A variety of lovers who will hold you, support you, and shape your growth. The ability to uncover new worlds of sexuality and play. *Yum yum yum yum yum!* But many people find the potential of discomfort is too much to bear. Feeling twinges of jealousy the first time you witness your partner kissing someone else. The uncertainty of allowing someone you love to act freely, hoping that they will have your best interests in mind. Having to spend a night alone when all of your other partners are busy with other obligations. *Ick ick ick ick ick!*

We withdraw from the *ick* faster than an amoeba can even swim. The fear of the *ick* drives people to hurriedly exclaim, "I could never be polyamorous. I'm way too much of a jealous person." It drives people to make these desperate attempts at controlling information, controlling their partner, or controlling the relationship. Relationship structure and agreements are formed with a focus on avoiding discomfort and pain at all costs, rather than on creating joy and pleasure. Whatever happens, no matter how good the *yum* is, it's not worth feeling all the *ick!*

Making the choice to embark on a journey of nontraditional romance means changing the way you see jealousy and fear. Instead of a shadowy source of dark feelings, it is a call to action. Instead of being dragons that need a prompt slaying, jealousy and fear are the tools that will crack your shell. And underneath that shell, you will see who you really are and what you really need. Your jealousy and fears are the X-ray the doctor orders to find out what's really going on inside to find the best way to heal it.

And so, if you're on the cusp of diving into polyamory or non-monogamy, it is imperative to accept the call to action. You need to choose to heal yourself, rather than protect yourself. You must choose to fuel your personal growth, rather than try to preserve yourself as you are right now. You have to choose changing yourself, changing your relationship, changing your paradigm, rather than stubbornly insisting that everything remain the same. Accepting this call to uncover yourself, having the courage to face the darkness within, and being willing to work on yourself frees you to enjoy all of the *yum* the world and the people you love have to offer.

Transforming Jealousy

This may all sound lovely and logical, but when your blood is boiling with jealousy or your stomach is twisting with fear over losing someone, logic only takes you so far. The process of transforming jealousy is different for everyone, and you may find that the most effective access point for you changes depending on the situation, the circumstances of your life, or what mood you wake up in on any given day.

Here are a number of tactics for approaching and transforming jealousy. This is far from a step-by-step list of instructions, though it may help to go through them in the order presented. Or you may find it better to pick and choose.

Let Yourself Feel It

Our inner amoeba wants to flee from unpleasant feelings, so it may seem counterintuitive to wallow in a self-made swamp of negative emotions. But letting yourself feel is different from wallowing. Here you're aiming to feel in such a way that you are able to deconstruct exactly what is going on inside when that big twinge of jealousy hits you. If you have meditation experience, this technique will be familiar.

When you are acutely aware of negative emotions coming up, find a quiet place where you'll be undisturbed, set a timer for ten minutes, and just sit with it. You don't have to be twisted up into lotus position, nor do you have to keep your eyes closed the whole time. During this time, instead of getting caught up in the maelstrom of thoughts in your head, bring your attention to how you actually feel. If you're experiencing jealousy, what lets you know that it is jealousy you're feeling? What are the physical characteristics of the feeling? There might be a tightening in your chest, or a fluttering sensation in the pit of your stomach, or a tingling in your hands. Get curious about these feelings, and really bring your focus to observing them. Avoid the temptation to analyze why or how they exist, and just watch what they do.

If you have a single-minded focus aimed at the feelings themselves, rather than on the thoughts and circumstances attached to them, it is likely that your emotional sensations will change or shift in some way. The tightening may switch to a pulsing, or it may feel more like a wave, or it may shift to another area of the body, and after a period of time it may disappear entirely!

This exercise helps us realize the transient nature of jealousy. Like every emotion, jealousy is ephemeral. The sensations of jealousy arise and pass, like every thought or feeling you've ever had. It is not a permanent state (thank goodness). Not even the most gut-wrenching, pulse-quickening wave of jealousy is immune to the old adage, "This too shall pass."

However, we are very good at getting in the way of this natural process of arising and passing. When jealous feelings arise, we either shy away and stuff them down in an attempt at ignoring them, or we stew in them, obsessively thinking about all the ways we've been wronged or how much we don't measure up. The irony is that both of these behaviors add fuel to the fire, making those unpleasant sensations last even longer. When you let yourself actually feel your emotions without attempting to squelch or bolster them, you'll be amazed how quickly they pass. Even in just ten minutes.

When your mind and body are clear and focused, no longer being tossed about by negative emotions, you are able to approach your partners, your situation, and your self with logic, compassion, and energy.

Change Your Emotional Frequency

It is imperative to separate your self—the self that produces results, communicates clearly and honestly, and deeply cares for others around you—from the constantly shifting landscape of your thoughts and feelings. When we're caught in negative emotions, it actually limits our cognitive ability to find creative solutions to problems, to think outside the box, or to look at things in a positive light. However, meditative approaches are not always accessible, especially if you've never tried any other kind of mindfulness work before or don't have the ability to step into a quiet, private space.

If being still or finding a quiet spot is not available to you, try swinging in the other direction. Engage in an activity that you know puts you in a good mood. For me, it's ecstatic dancing. I put on upbeat music and just move in whatever way feels good, maybe including some off-key singing if the mood strikes. If I'm in the car at the time, this involves a lot of steering wheel percussion and shoulder shimmies. For others this may be going for a run, playing a co-op video game with your best friend, watching your favorite stand-up comedian, reading an inspirational book, or indulging in some guilty-pleasure fast food.

However, it's important to make sure this doesn't turn into a habit of mindlessly distracting or numbing yourself. After about thirty minutes to an hour of engaging in your mood-lifting activity, check in with yourself. Check what you're feeling, what you're thinking about, and if there are any new perspectives or insights surrounding the situation that triggered your jealousy. Chances are you'll be able to think clearly, feel more positively, and communicate in a way that is effective and compassionate.

Write It Out

Writing is often lauded as an excellent outlet for taming scattered thoughts and feelings. You might find great emotional release in unstructured writing, letting your stream of consciousness flow across the page so that it's no longer plaguing your mind. This "writing dump" might turn into an elaborate piece of prose, or a letter to someone, or a cathartic poem. It may end up being more raw as well ("FUCK FUCK FUCK" written across the page in red marker, as the authors of *The Ethical Slut* suggest).[5]

Structured writing is also useful to put together the puzzle pieces of what you're feeling and how to cope with it. Psychotherapist Jennice Vilhauer recommends this particular exercise for assuring and supporting yourself through tough emotions and negative thoughts.

First, think about what you fear will happen. Then, write down all the reasons why that thing will not happen. As Vilhauer points out, most of the things we worry about don't actually come to pass![6] For example, your fear might be:

My wife is going to leave me for someone better than me.

The list of reasons why that is unlikely to happen might look like this:

We've been together for over five years now, and our bond is strong, healthy, and irreplaceable.
We are great communicators, unafraid to tell each other the truth about what we're feeling.
My wife constantly tells me how much she loves me, and how much she loves planning for the future with me.

The human brain is skilled at finding evidence to support our fears and insecurities, but often we overlook all of the evidence to the contrary. Writing out all the reasons why you actually are safe, secure, and happy can help put you in a mindset of abundance and plenty, rather than one of lack and insecurity.

The second part of the writing exercise is to write down why you would still be okay, even if your worst fears were to happen. This is the place to focus on your strengths, the things that make you unique, and the inner qualities that have gotten you through rough times in the past. Instead of focusing on how broken and devastated you might be if things don't turn out the way you want, it is self-affirming to focus on the confidence that you have to get through it. Your list might look something like this:

I have a wide network of loving family and friends who are there to support me emotionally. I've always been good at maintaining a positive attitude, even when I'm under stress. All of the difficult times in my life have resulted in so much personal growth and gaining valuable life lessons. I don't regret any of it, because I learned so much.

Pay It Forward

A long time ago, someone once told me, "If you feel like you need love, go out and give love to somebody." It sounds trite and overly simple, but it's stuck with me for years. I didn't really puzzle over the meaning of it, or how it might work, until I started experiencing jealousy in one of my relationships.

I was sitting alone one night while one of my partners was spending time with another girl. She was someone that I didn't particularly care for, and I was stewing in my own mess of jealousy, insecurity, and overall ickiness. All I could think about was how I wasn't getting what I wanted. I wanted attention, I wanted affection, I wanted love, and there was no one there to give it to me. Poor me.

I remembered that piece of advice, and even though I didn't feel like I had anything to give, I gave it a try. Even though he was busy with his date, I sent a text message to my partner about how much I appreciated him. I knew I wouldn't get a response for a few hours, but sitting there with the phone in my hand, I noticed that I did feel a little bit better. Encouraged, I also sent a message to another partner, complimenting him on how sexy he looked when I last saw him. I definitely felt much more positive now, and I called up my sister to tell her how much I missed her and ask about what was going on in her life. Our conversation was brief, but afterward I felt content, peaceful, and full of love. I've been hooked on this technique ever since.

If you're struggling with jealousy, the mind wants to focus on all the things that you're not getting. It wants to obsess over what is making you feel bad, all the ways that you are inadequate, and how sad and pathetic your situation is. You may even be tempted to reach out to other people in a needy, attention-seeking manner. But in putting the focus outside of yourself, in extending positivity and love to someone else with no expectation of anything in return, there's an internal shift. You are able move past the doubt, the cold, the darkness, and invite in warmth, positivity, and love. It's the easiest quick fix for jealous feelings that I've found to date.

Talk About It

You guessed it: communication is the answer, once again. Though transforming jealousy is mostly an internal process, there is much to be gained by sharing it with others. If a brilliant insight arose while meditating on your feelings, or if you've gained some new perspective on how great your relationships are after writing about their individual strengths, take the opportunity to share that knowledge with your partners. It can be embarrassing to own up to moments of jealousy, insecurity, and vulnerability, but sharing the lessons and insights you've gained with your partners allows them to understand even more of you and what makes you tick.

Sometimes, just a few words of reassurance can help eliminate inner turmoil. It can be as simple as saying to your partner, "I'm feeling a little insecure. Can you tell me that you love me and that there's nothing for me to worry about?" This should be easy for your partner to give. If you know that hearing your partner say something in particular or having a certain conversation will alleviate your fears, then have no hesitations in requesting it!

More Thoughts on Jealousy

❝My advice, if you can understand and accept this one statement, then any gender can be in a poly relationship, and that is: 'I understand that your (your partner's) love for someone else does not affect your love for me.' That one statement has gotten me through any and every bout of jealousy, though they have been few and far between.❞ —Julie

❝Jealousy is not a be-all, end-all to things. You can work through your emotions to find the positive feelings in seeing your partner happy; it can take time, but it can get easier.❞ —Bria

❝Treat jealousy as a symptom of an underlying issue, then go after that issue, delight in the joy of your partners, and love, love, love before all else.❞ —Rebecca

Chapter 5 Homework

Exercise #1

Remember a time when you felt jealous of someone who wasn't a romantic partner, such as a friend, family member, or coworker. What techniques did you use to cope with the feelings of jealousy? Would any of those techniques apply to romantic or sexual jealousy?

Exercise #2

When you are experiencing twinges of jealousy, try changing your perspective on yourself. Visualize what the situation would be like if the circumstances were exactly the same (your partner is going on a date, or sharing a new experience with another partner, or whatever may be triggering you). The only difference is to imagine the situation and pretend that you feel completely self-confident, assured, secure, and happy with yourself. Would you still feel jealous or threatened?

The next time your jealousy is triggered, try making a proactive choice to act self-confident, self-loving, and secure, even if you feel like you are faking it. Take note if the situation that triggers your jealousy still feels as scary or unmanageable.

6 The Second Biggest Question: Sex

American culture in particular can't seem to really decide what sex is or how to feel about it. When I was growing up in a religious household, sex was a sacred covenant, a precious bond of intimacy so special that it had to be saved and given only to my future husband. After I actually had sex for the first time (not with my future husband), sex became a comfortably normal, human process, much like eating or sweating or going to the bathroom. Pickup artist books and websites would have you believe that sex is the be-all and end-all, and to the man with the highest number go the spoils. Certain high school textbooks claim that sex is a perilous landscape of diseases and unwanted pregnancy, avoidable only by keeping your legs firmly shut.

My own generation of millennials grew up with unfettered access to the world of Internet erotica, an intense and arguably unnatural first introduction to sex. Scientists and journalists shine light on pornography and sex addiction, endlessly questioning if such a thing is normal, aberrant, shameful, or if we can even properly use the word "addiction" at all. We consume copious amounts of sexual content, via porn aggregates, webcam sites, and even blockbuster films. Yet we have a difficult time discussing or envisioning sex that falls outside of the hyper-romantic sheen of the movies or the fervent mash-cut overload of pornography. And God forbid you openly talk about sex if you're disabled, or overweight, or elderly, or if your genitals don't quite fit into either Gender A or Gender B.

In the middle of this tangled nest of sexual confusion lie polyamory and non-monogamy. If the number one question is jealousy, the number two question is inevitably about sex. *Don't you feel weird about your partners all having sex with someone else? Aren't you scared of catching a disease? Do you have group sex all the time?*

Leaders in the polyamory scene do their best to allay the assumption that this lifestyle is all about sex. We talk a lot about how important it is to focus on building healthy, meaningful relationships, and that it's all about sharing an abundance of love. This is true, but at the end of the day, sex is still a very important point of discussion in non-monogamous relationships, whether you're bursting with high libido or happily asexual. This chapter will examine exactly where polyamory lies within that discussion and negotiation, as well as covering the most important things you need to know about communication, risk, and the wide, teeming world of sexual exploration.

Transforming Sex Negativity

Few of us feel totally comfortable making a no-questions-asked, head-first dive into sexual exploration. Sometimes getting yourself, your partners, or your friends to talk openly, honestly, and unabashedly about sex can be like pulling teeth. Even if you were to openly discuss these things, would that count as sharing too much information? Will someone get offended? How do I even talk about sex acts and body parts without either sounding like Dr. Ruth or a middle schooler?

These thoughts and feelings may be familiar to you if you grew up in a sex-negative environment. This environment could be bred by the religion you grew up with, a conservative political climate, the attitudes of your parents, or the culture at large. As you'll remember from the discussion in chapter 1 on slut-shaming and the Madonna-whore complex, it's not just polyamorous women who get caught in the cross fire of sex negativity, but everyone. Even though my generation of peers has better access to sexual education, birth control, and sexual healthcare than generations past, we are still struggling to cast off centuries of sexual shame.

Many sexually active women, including myself, have still inwardly cringed upon revealing to someone their number of past sex partners. And so I, like so many other women, shrink from the conversation itself. Whether your all-important number is three hundred or three, someone is going to think that it's far too many. Slut-shaming is real and potently affects the lives of every woman who is sexually active (and often those who are not as well). How do we combat this? What needs to happen in order to become a fully alive, comfortable, whole, and complete sexual being, free of guilt or shame?

Large-scale shifts in cultural attitudes may seem daunting and unattainable, but they are necessary, and they begin on the individual level. Sex-negative attitudes are transformed by educating yourself about sexual health and sexual communities other than your own. These attitudes can also be reshaped by sexual exploration itself—by expanding your horizons, learning about new techniques, and uncovering new desires. Do not underestimate the power of taking ownership of your sexual needs, wants, and interests, and having no fear or shame in pursuing sexual fulfillment. Remember, you get to define what your sex life is; it does not get to define you. Because, thankfully, you are far more than your body parts, your fetishes, your sexual preferences, or your number of sex partners, past and present.

Sex and the Polyamorous Woman

Sex negativity clashes pretty hard with the ideals of being in a non-monogamous relationship. If you are open with people about having more than one partner, chances are they will take it as a clear announcement that you're bangin' more than one person (even if not all of your relationships are sexual in nature). Seeing a woman indirectly indicate an interest in sex, and sex with multiple people at that, is enough to turn heads. This can result in the assumption that any polyamorous woman must have an insatiable sexual appetite and be willing to hop into bed with anyone and everyone who crosses her path. This assumption either leads to copious amounts of unwanted attention or, at worst, the condemnation, vilification, and criticism inherent in slut-shaming. More on this in chapter 11.

In a culture of slut-shaming, the number of sexual partners you've had over the course of your lifetime carries weight. The unfortunate reality is that what counts as "too much" or "too few" is different for everyone. To you, this number may represent a colorful history of intimate connections and playful evenings, each unique and memorable in their own right. But to others, this number may represent proof that you are used up, slovenly, careless, possibly dirty, and diseased. A woman who has had two sex partners in the past will be rejected by some people, while other people would think she was too innocent and inexperienced, while others wouldn't really give a hoot. Even tallying up your number comes with problems: what makes it onto the list? Is it just the people you've had penetrative sex with? What if the sex you have doesn't involve penetration at all?

Numbers and Meaning

It's important to be up-front about your sexual history for reasons of health and safety, but it is also a shared responsibility to combat assumptions that a woman who has had multiple sex partners is used up or dirty. Remember that regardless of what a person's number may be, it doesn't mean anything about who he or she is in this very moment. If you find yourself uncomfortable with your own sexual history, or with a partner's sexual history, take time to examine the origins of those feelings. Do they come from expectations and assumptions inherited from your culture, religion, upbringing, or the reactions of others?

Dirty Words

Sex negativity is so ingrained in Western culture that it is even built into the English language. Many of the words used as expletives are sex acts, body parts, or bodily functions: fuck, tits, cock, cunt, etc. In our everyday language, we associate sexual terminology with wrongdoing, dirtiness, and negativity. Strangely, the truly dark and harmful aspects of human behavior (murder, rape, hatred, torture, etc.) are not considered dirty words. Something to think about.

Sex and Definitions of Sex

Sex, much like spirituality, is a personal journey. Each encounter and interaction serves to shape your own unique definition of sexuality, from when you were a kid playing doctor to losing your virginity to the first time you experimented with something kinky and new. What sex means to you is different from what it means to your next-door neighbor. You've already answered a number of questions about sex from chapter 3, but now is the time to dig a little deeper into the intricacies of your inner sexual being.

The seemingly obvious fundamentals of sex are ripe for questioning. Is sex just penetration? For anyone who has had sex with men, women, and individuals outside of the gender binary, it is patently clear that sex can be defined far beyond the simple act of a penis entering a vagina. What about figuring out when sex has actually begun? Is it when you've touched another person's genitalia, when you've taken off clothes, or did it start from the moment you shared a glance across the room? And how do you know when sex ends? Is it after everyone has had an orgasm? Or is it only over once you're too exhausted to keep going? The answers to these questions will be different for each person, and not everyone will follow the "standard" format for vanilla heterosexual sex. (Usually kissing, then foreplay, then penetrative sex until one or both parties have had an orgasm.) Even beyond figuring out your personal definition of sex, it's important to know what *good* sex is to you, which is a whole other exploration entirely.

Good, Good Sex

Because of the pervasive nature of sex negativity, many of us are internally cut off from our sexual desires. Not only is sex tied up with shame, dirtiness, and sin, but on the flip side, we are taught very clearly who it is that we *should* find sexy and what "good sex" is supposed to look like. Tall, rugged men with washboard abs, women with overspilling cleavage, leather high-heeled boots, and a duvet covered in rose petals, seen through the Vaseline-covered camera lens associated with softcore porn and Barbra Streisand.

However, good sex is made up of many moving parts. Good sex is not only physically pleasurable, but mentally and emotionally as well. It lets you express yourself, either just as you are, warts and all, or as you are in the realm of fantasy (the ravenous, conquering Amazon or the treasured yet rebellious slave-in-training come to mind). It lets us explore the body and soul connection between people, whether it's your lover of twenty years, or the person you just met at a play party. Your version of good sex may involve several orgasms or none. It could involve multiple people at the same time, or just yourself. It could be solidly vanilla or no-holds-barred, unabashedly weird and kinky. Jessica Graham, author of *Good Sex: Getting Off Without Checking Out*, puts it well:

> **"**Good Sex allows for evolution and flexibility. Humans are amazing creatures and what turns us on and gets us off can change many times throughout a life. Good Sex requires us to be willing to look with eyes wide open at our shadow self, our trauma, and

our ingrained beliefs. Good Sex is neither being attached or indifferent. It is being fully present, without grasping, for the amazing thing that happens when people decide to come together to do what we have been doing since the beginning of humankind. And Good Sex is hot as hell, let's not forget that."[1]

You may be quite certain of what makes good sex for you, or you could be totally clueless! If you are totally clueless, how do you discover what it is you want? And if you're already quite sure of what it is you like, how do you expand yourself and learn more?

Different Libidos, Different Desires

Though some people come to alternative relationships because of a voracious libido, it is far from a universal motivation. People with low libidos or who are completely asexual often find non-monogamy to be a perfect fit, as it allows their partners to find sexual satisfaction from other places, without having to sacrifice their relationships. Others find that they don't need a higher or lower frequency of sex, but rather enjoy having a variety of different partners, each bringing unique personalities, body types, sexual techniques, and desires. Still other people choose to involve themselves with multiple others because of a particular fetish. If you get all hot and bothered by the idea of totally dominating someone, but your current partner has zero interest in being submissive, you can still scratch that itch by having the ability and opportunity to find someone whose lifelong dream has been to be tied up, tickled, teased, and pleased, all under your command.

Self Love and Sexploration

The first step is in learning what feels good when you are by yourself. Masturbation can be not only an important aspect of self-care, but yet another means of getting to know yourself physically, emotionally, and mentally. Fortunately, the taboo surrounding female masturbation is dissipating, though studies show that men still masturbate significantly more often than women do.[2]

This is unsurprising when most masturbatory material is produced for men. Advertisements, movies, and pornography are usually shot with the male gaze in mind, heavily featuring the body parts of the female actress, with her male counterpart's head and face and sometimes entire body cropped out of the frame. Pornography and erotica packaged for women are either tongue-in-cheek (a book of images featuring men doing housework) or re-branded gay porn (rippling, oiled-up beefcakes in tiny underwear). Many people attribute this to the fact that women are just not visually aroused, a callback to the results of Kinsey's studies on sexuality in the 1950s.[3] Contemporary research and observation of brainwave frequencies find that women experience just as quick and enthusiastic a response to erotic images as men do.[4] In this case, nurture, rather than nature, has trained women to abstain from consuming the same amounts of pornography as the average male. The relative dearth of erotic material for women seems to imply that women do not and should not seek arousing media, nor strive to pleasure themselves.

Regardless of a lack of mainstream support, exploring one's body, sexuality, and arousal is illuminating. Whether you are quite confident in your self-pleasuring or you are only just beginning to explore yourself, it is useful to take a "beginner's mind" approach. This means letting go of the things that you think you already know about yourself as a sexual being. You may have particular fantasies, fetishes, or an extremely specific way of masturbating every time. It's challenging, but see if you can play a game with yourself: if you shook the Etch-A-Sketch of your sexual makeup, what new or different things could you try?

This is a useful technique for distinguishing which things actually turn you on and get you off, and which things are inherited from culture, media, or your peer group. When I was a teenager, I learned masturbation technique from watching mainstream pornography. There was plenty of study material on the Internet, but I found that no matter how closely I copied what I watched, I could not have an orgasm. This continued for five or six years, and at the age of eighteen I internally accepted that I might be one of those women who just never have an orgasm. Imagine my confusion and delight when my very first orgasm caught me totally by surprise in the middle of intercourse, and it dawned on me that in all my years of frustrated masturbation, doing everything that I thought I was supposed to do, I'd never tried to find what actually felt good to me. I've heard from one woman who was completely restrained in the whole BDSM works—handcuffs, leg spreader, ball-gag, etc.—when she realized that she didn't get any pleasure from being bound up. She had gotten caught up in the fervor of all of her girlfriends reading *50 Shades of Grey*, and thrown herself into the world of BDSM mostly because everyone else seemed to be doing it. This woman later did happily return to her explorations of bondage . . . but as the one doing the tying instead.

It is necessary to let go of preconceived or culturally installed ideas of what you *should* find sexy in order to discover what you actually *do* find sexy. This requires bringing mindfulness to your brain and body and being vigilant in noticing the sights, sounds, smells, and situations that get your nerves tingling and whisks your mind into the realm of tempting fantasy, whether for a brief moment or for the rest of the day. These may be surprisingly random things: seeing the way your lover adjusts her glasses, the growling quality in your boyfriend's voice when he's waking up in the morning, seeing anyone who is smartly dressed in suspenders. (That last one is entirely my own. Don't ask me to explain.)

On the physical side, this means some exploratory self-pleasuring. (I know, it's a chore, but someone's gotta do it.) You may try slowing things down, setting aside time to focus on just experiencing pleasure, rather than racing toward orgasm as quickly as possible. If you always masturbate in the same position with the same technique, try switching it up. Get yourself aroused in one position, then bring yourself to orgasm in an entirely different position. Changing your self-love routine expands your sexual versatility, which positively affects your partnered sex life as well.

Pornography

We've come a long way from the days of crumpled-up nudie mags and late-night skin flicks on cable TV. Now, porn is accessible nearly at the speed of thought. Heterosexual men have the widest variety of options available, but there's a growing market for every sexuality, gender identity, and crazy, off-the-wall fetish you could think of.

Porn and the porn industry is a mixed bag. On the one hand, there's no denying the copious amounts of pornographic content that is degrading, insensitive, unrealistic, and downright abusive. There are now multiple generations of children and teenagers whose first exposure to sex is the hyper-stimulating world of Internet pornography. In the absence of universally accessible, comprehensive sex education, many people grow up with pornography as their only source of information on sex and sexuality. Imagine learning how to drive when your only educational resource is the *Fast and the Furious* film franchise.

On the other hand, there's a reason why porn is so popular. A large proportion of the human race enjoys watching other members of the human race having sex. Maybe it harks back to the days of living in tribes, where privacy wasn't a given. Maybe seeing other people have sex meant that things are good: the tribe is safe, fed, having fun, and hey, maybe I'll get to join in! Whatever the reason, we did not evolve to be instinctually disgusted by sex or repulsed by others having sex. If we were, that'd be the end of the road for our species pretty quickly.

If you are not actively involved in a swinging or sex party community, you may not have frequent opportunities to watch other people having sex outside of the realm of pornography. But there isn't anything inherently wrong in wanting to take in sexual imagery. It is your decision to determine how pornography may or may not fit into your life. As with many things in life, seek moderation and mindfulness. Moderation in porn consumption will protect against desensitization, or ending up in a rut where you are unable to become aroused during sex with a partner. Mindfulness will help you examine the kinds of erotic imagery you choose to consume, or what things you might want to share with your partners.

Expanding Your Sexual Landscape

Most people find their sexual spectrum widens with exposure to their partner's desires, preferences, and fetishes. If you have multiple sexual partners, you will quickly find a vastly different array of kinks and quirks, ranging from vanilla to the unconventional. It is best to err on the side of saying yes to exploring your partner's kinks rather than no, unless his or her kinks directly violate a personal boundary. Allow yourself to be surprised by discovering new things, including things you previously thought were not for you.

Your partner may approach you with a fetish, fantasy, or particular form of sex play that you have never tried before. Remember that being privy to someone's inmost sexual desires is a great privilege, and her vulnerability should be respected accordingly. If you are unsure about your partner's interests, do your research before giving a flat-out "no." The best way I've found to do this is to find some written erotica that primarily focuses on the fetish in question. While pornography may quite clearly (and bombastically) offer a visual demonstration of a particular fantasy, well-written erotica gives you a glimpse into the psychology behind it. You get to step into the mind of someone already experiencing this fantasy; you become wise to what makes the physical sensations appealing and the thought process that heightens the situation to the level of sexual excitement. You may even ask your partner to find an erotic story that particularly resonates with her, and then send it to you to read. The reverse of this is also useful if you are the one who has a particular fetish that you want to share with a partner.

Sexuality and Fluidity

Sexual exploration involves not just trying out new positions or adventurous fantasies, but examining the landscape of your sexuality as well. Sexual orientation is far from the clear-cut black and white that most of us have been taught. We are used to envisioning a spectrum: heterosexuality on one end, homosexuality on the other. In theory, everyone falls at some point on this spectrum; some closer to the middle, and some closer to either end. However, I would propose throwing this image out the window. Instead of a solid line demarcated with degrees of "straightness" or "gayness," imagine more of an intricate yet chaotic, Pollock-esque web. There are no extremes on a spectrum, but floating vertices in a wide network of qualities, genders, emotions, and sexual desires.

It is difficult to apply a simple label to such a complex thing as human sexuality. I have had sex with both men and women, and my preference skews toward men. I hold less of a sexual attraction to women, but I'm still romantically attracted to women—I'm more excited by the idea of holding, kissing, cuddling, and caressing a woman than having intercourse with her. Some people prefer having sex with a particular gender, but find that they experience sexual attraction to the other gender after developing a close emotional bond. Does that still count as bisexual? What about the woman dating a cisgender man who spends most of his time dressing as a woman? Does that make her straight? Gay? Somewhere in between?

If you have never examined or questioned your sexual orientation before, it is an illuminating exercise to really look at why you are the way you are—even if you feel comfortable and solid in your sexuality, even if you feel sure that there's no way it could change. The awesome thing about polyamory is that it enables you to explore all kinds of relationships with all kinds of sexual expression and orientations outside of hetero- or homosexuality. Let's briefly cover a few of the most common labels, though remember that this is far from an extensive list.

asexual—Does not experience sexual attraction or strong desires for sex, but may still desire romantic and emotionally involved relationships.[5]
aromantic—Experiences very little to no romantic attraction to other people. May still experience sexual desire, but will often find satisfaction in friendships or other non-romantic interactions.[6]
bisexual or biromantic—Experiences attraction to both men and women. This attraction may be sexual, romantic, or both. Some people experience sexual attraction to both sexes, but only feel romantic attraction for one sex, and vice versa.
pansexual—Sexually or romantically attracted to all gender identities. May also refer to a person whose sexual identity and attraction is fluid.[7]
demisexual—Only experiences sexual attraction to a person after forming a close or familiar bond with them.[8]
demiromantic—Also known as "gray romantic." Only experiences romantic attraction to a person after forming a close or familiar bond with them.[9]
hetero- or homoflexible—Identifies primarily as heterosexual or as homosexual, yet under certain circumstances may choose to engage with members of whichever sex is outside of their usual preference.

Aromanticism and Asexuality

An *aromantic* person is someone who feels very little or no romantic attraction to other people. Aromantics need support and care, like all human beings, but generally these needs are met by healthy relationships with family and friends. An aromantic person may still feel sexual attraction and be physically affectionate to others, but she may rarely or never experience any feelings of falling in love or hold any desire to be in a romantic relationship. Instead having of a crush, she may have a "friend crush" or a "squish"—a strong desire to develop a platonic relationship with someone.

Along the same vein, an *asexual* person is someone who feels little or no sexual attraction to others. Asexuality may be considered a part of a person's inherent sexuality, as opposed to people who elect celibacy or abstinence. An asexual person may still desire romantic connection, and she may still experience sexual arousal, but neither of these feelings preclude a desire for any kind of sexual relationship.

Aromantics and asexuals do exist, but they are often misunderstood in a culture where romantic love is put on a pedestal, and where sex is consistently marketed as the best thing since sliced bread. There are also some who identify as demiromantic or demisexual, meaning they only experience romantic or sexual attraction (respectively) after they have formed a close emotional bond with another person. Some people, like Catherine, experience a switch from one to the other:

"*I identified as strictly asexual for my entire life until I met Daniel and found that I had a whole new side of me that needed expressing. However, romance does not express itself to me sexually. The sex I do have is less an expression of love and romance and more like an extra activity I get to take part in. A lot of people just view demisexual as a label for having standards and waiting. Genuinely though, it's the fact that sexual attraction to a person for me does not exist without friendship and a strong platonic base, and even after that it is still highly likely that it won't be there.***"** —Catherine

A Word on Bisexuality

The term "bisexual" is common knowledge, but its meaning is deceptively simple. It just means someone who is attracted to both sexes, right? In reality, there is a wealth of different meanings and interpretations, and some people eschew the label altogether as it implies that only two sexes exist. Some people choose the term based on their orientation of being attracted to both, others based on their actual practice of sexually engaging with both sexes. However, there is a wide difference in how bisexuality is viewed depending on what your sex is.

Female-female relationships suffer from a lack of perceived weight and meaning. Girls will get drunk and make out in a bar for the entertainment of the male patrons; so-called lesbian pornography is largely created with the male viewer in mind and rarely enacted by women who actually identify as lesbian. There's a cultural acceptance of women partaking in this kind of college-age, experimental "girlish fun." Some women even feel obligated to engage in bisexual activity, either because everyone else seems to be doing it, or because it elicits a positive response from men. This phenomenon may elicit the opposite response as well: causing truly bisexual women to shy away from female-female relationships because of the perception that they are fleeting and meaningless.

On the other hand, male-male relationships are crushed under the burden of far too much meaning. Bisexual men are pariahs. The general consensus from heterosexuals is that bisexual men are just too afraid to fully come out of the closet as gay, and the homosexual community accuses bisexual men of wanting to get their rocks off without the full brunt of social stigma that comes with being gay. You'll find a consensus among many women who feel uncomfortable thinking about their male partner engaging in any kind of homosexual activity, either due to the perception that this hobbles his masculinity, or that he secretly is more fulfilled by being with men than with women.

As mentioned above, sexuality is a web rather than a spectrum. I have met several women who desire a lifelong, shared-bank-account-and-raising-kids romantic partnership with women, but still have sexual desire for men. And I've met several men who love the idea of holding hands, kissing, and dating other men, but who are not aroused by the thought of sex with a man. (This sentiment is also common in reverse!)

Many people abandon the label of "bisexual" because it is too simplistic and reductive. Instead, some choose to describe their complex sexuality in great detail: "I have dated both women and men, but I have a preference for men romantically and for women sexually," for example. And some choose instead to adopt the label of "pansexual," accounting for attraction to everyone who falls outside of the male-female gender binary, such as genderqueer, intersex, or trans folk.

Kinky Love

There has long been an overlap between the poly community and the kink community. Many people choose to incorporate kink and sexuality into their relationship structures, monogamously or non-monogamously. There are many different relationship formats, but two of the most common in poly circles are Dom/sub relationships and cuckold/cuckquean relationships.

D/s relationships are characterized by one partner acting as the dominant, while the other acts as the submissive. While some people only explore this power play in the bedroom or at BDSM clubs, others choose to incorporate it into their relationship structure as a whole. The Dom may control aspects of the sub's life, including how the sub dresses and who the sub is allowed to play with. Some people may engage in a D/s relationship with one partner, but have "vanilla" relationships with all other partners. Others may find themselves sub to multiple Doms, or vice versa!

Cuckold/cuckqueans get off on seeing their partner have sex with other people, but not necessarily for the sake of voyeurism. Cuckolds and cuckqueans derive pleasure from their partner consensually "cheating" on them for a variety of reasons—knowing that their partner is attractive and desired by others, or through eroticized feelings of humiliation. Cuckolds and cuckqueans may choose to take this fantasy outside of the realm of sexual play, and allow their partner to pursue outside relationships. The cuckold/cuckquean may choose to remain monogamous.

The combination of kink and poly raises questions of ethics. If a Dom commands that her sub must remain monogamous, while the Dom herself is allowed to have many subs and partners, is that really fair? If a cuckquean chooses to remain monogamous while her partner sleeps around, does she have any right to complain about feeling jealous or left out?

Bending the traditional rules of relationships can be great fun romantically and sexually, but take care that the format of the relationship doesn't overrule the feelings and needs of the people in the relationship. Even though a sub agrees to give up some of his control and autonomy to a Dom, he is still a decision-maker in the relationship. Although a cuckold may enjoy his partner's wanton behavior, he still needs emotional and sexual care of his own. By all means, go out and have kinky sex and kinky relationships if it floats your boat, but only if it's bringing joy and satisfaction to everyone involved.

Group Sex

Inevitably, someone will ask you if polyamory means having orgies all the time. I usually counter this question by asking if monogamy means having sex all the time. For some people, a monogamous relationship may be characterized by frequent sex; for others there may be no sex at all. It's the same with polyamorous people and group sex. For the purpose of this discussion, the term "group sex" covers any sexual interaction involving more than two people, from a threesome all the way to an elaborately orchestrated orgy at a sex party.

Any given person in a polyamorous community may have zero interest in having more than two people in a sexual interaction, and another person may be tumbling around in sexy puppy piles every weekend. It all depends on each individual's preferences; however, the polyamorous community does seem to be more conducive to these kinds of sexual interactions taking place, compared to monogamous communities. Participating in group sex requires a certain level of sex positivity, adventurousness, open-mindedness, and a dash of kinkiness as well.

Group sex captures the imaginations of many, partly due to the fact that it scratches many itches that are still taboo. You can experience the thrill of the voyeur, watching other people interact and getting full access to something that would normally be hidden away. Simultaneously you can feel the rush of being an exhibitionist, feeling the excitement of other eyes watching, of other minds and bodies getting excited by observing you. And your world can be totally rocked by the sensory overload of being touched and pleasured by a variety of people at the same time.

Just like two-person sex, group sex can be either a casual romp with the sole purpose of naughty fun, or it can be an intimate exploration of the sexual chemistry and mysterious dynamics only present among a particular set of people. If you have an interest in exploring group sex, it is important to ask yourself which aspect is most appealing to you.

If you want to fulfill some fantasies and dive into the purely recreational side of group sex, it's easiest to connect with a swinger's community or to vet some sex clubs or resorts in your area. If you show yourself to be respectful, a good communicator, and a positive presence, it should be relatively easy to find other like-minded people who want to have sexy fun and help bring your sultry fantasies to life.

If you are more drawn to exploring the intimate side of group sex, it requires the patience and flexibility to let your exploration be organic. If you find that your partner's other partner is alluring, intriguing, and you could see yourself dating this person, why not take a crack at it! Worst-case scenario, the two of you go on a date and find that there isn't actually any chemistry and things stay mostly the way they were; best-case scenario, you have the grounds for a happy and healthy triad relationship, with the potential for all kinds of sexy times together. You also may find yourself connected to a network of sexually open poly relationships and close friendships, making it much easier for everyone to click and come together for some orgiastic play. (Although past experience has taught me that trying to coordinate multiple schedules for this sort of thing is a feat in itself.) Before you get too excited by the possibilities, remember that you are neither obligated nor entitled to play with any of your partner's other partners, and your partner is neither obligated nor entitled to play with any of yours. Be sure to check in and confirm that everyone who is joining your group play has consented to it.

Problems arise when group sex is pursued via the wrong avenues. If you want to have close, intimate sex with multiple people that you know and love, you may come out of a swinger's party feeling like a piece of meat—used only for a night of fun and not even a phone call afterward. If you seek out a committed triad relationship primarily in the hopes that you'll get to fulfill a lifelong fantasy of having threesomes, you may unintentionally hurt someone when his or her expectations for investment and emotional care are not met.

So You're About to Have Group Sex

Congratulations! You're getting to have an experience that much of the population only gets to fantasize about. Important things to keep in mind:

- Give your consent to everyone involved, and make sure everyone else is consenting as well.
- Communicate often. Check in frequently to make sure everyone feels happy and safe. If you or someone else is not feeling comfortable, do not hesitate to pause and talk about what needs to change in order to get everyone on the same page. If someone needs to stop, give nothing but compassion and understanding. Avoid judgment, shaming, guilt, or coercion.
- Make sure everyone is in agreement about safe sex practices. If you've all agreed on using barriers, bring plenty of them. If you are using condoms, remember that a new condom needs to be used with each partner.
- Bring lots of lubricant.
- Stay hydrated by having plenty of water on hand. If you drink alcohol, one drink may be helpful to relax nerves, but imbibing too much will dehydrate you and limit your ability to give full consent or feedback.
- Have fun!

STIs and Sexual Risk

No discussion on sex would be complete without talking about sexual health. All sex has some form of risk, just as crossing the street, diving into a pool, and getting out of bed in the morning have some form of risk. The only way to completely avoid any of the risks of sex is to avoid having it completely. However, for those of us to whom the risks of sex are not a total deal breaker, there are plenty of ways to mitigate them.

Adding more sex partners increases your chances of being exposed to STIs. This doesn't mean that you have to approach every sexual encounter in a hazmat suit, but it does mean that you need to define what "safer sex" means to you and discuss it with your partners. Some people will choose to only engage in "dry" sex that has no fluid contact or transmission whatsoever. Others will engage in fluid transmission, but maintain complete coverage of any areas exposed—that means dental dams, condoms for penetrative and oral sex, rubber gloves, etc. Still others will choose to have fully unprotected sex with one or multiple partners, provided everyone is informed, tested, and has agreed to this.

If you are engaging in heterosexual activity, it is imperative to plan for some kind of birth control method, unless you are willingly trying to conceive a child. Both STI prevention and contraception are shared responsibilities, but be sure that you are looking out for yourself first and foremost. This means taking the reins on choosing the kind of protection that makes you feel the safest, communicating about it with your partners, and having a backup method.

There is a wealth of information, facts, and figures on every STI and birth control technology under the sun. Unfortunately, sexual health has been tightly entwined with politics and religious expression. As such, some information resources may manipulate, skew, edit, or alter facts in order to support a particular bias or stance. Do your own research, seek information from multiple credible sources, and always check your facts. You can find links to the most reliable STI and sexual health information in the Resources section.

Sexual Stigma

People living with STIs often face harsh negative reactions. We rarely judge someone when they pick up any other kind of infection: the common cold, hepatitis, or the flu. But because sex-negative cultures already associate sex with being dirty and shameful, any infection that is the result of sexual contact is even more damning. Even STIs that do not carry the immediate risk of debilitating illness or death, such as herpes simplex (HSV-1 and HSV-2), still come with the weight of a derogatory reputation.

If your partner or metamour tests positive for an STI, always choose to educate yourself first before leveling judgment or blame. Find reliable information, then take whatever actions you need in order to keep yourself and your partners healthy and safe. If you have tested positive for an STI, you should not only educate yourself, but prepare to educate the other people you are sexual with. Having your facts straight is an excellent way to preclude assumptions and misinformed decisions.

Barriers and Intimacy

Some polyamorists choose to engage in "fluid bonding." This refers to people who have chosen to have fully unprotected sex with each other, usually after STI testing and establishing reliable birth control. Some people choose to do this with only one person; some choose to do so with multiple people. I avoid using the term "fluid bonding," as the phrase perpetuates a common societal quirk: associating unbarriered sex with intimacy.

It makes perfect sense why we see unbarriered sex as being more intimate. In many traditional monogamous relationships, having sex without a condom or dental dam is a milestone. It signifies that you've foregone having sex with anyone else, that you've chosen to trust each other, that you're removing all literal and figurative barriers between you. In a heterosexual marriage, it may signify the moment when the couple decides to conceive a baby. There is a lot of importance attached to it.

Conversely, this attaches some negativity to protected sex. Some people see condom or dental dam usage as a sign of mistrust or that the relationship is not important or meaningful. People practicing hierarchical polyamory may deem the primary relationship as the only one special enough to merit unprotected sex, with all secondary partners kept quite literally behind a barrier that prevents them from getting "too" intimate.

It's time for a reality check. Condoms and dental dams are not magical intimacy-blocking force fields, nor are they beacons of shame and mistrust. They are nothing more than bits of latex. They are quite useful for preventing exposure to certain bacteria and viruses, as well as containing rogue genetic material hell-bent on making babies. Any other meaning attached to its presence or absence is personal interpretation. Your decision to use protection has nothing to do with your partner, or with your partner's partners. It only has to do with you making the decision to take care of your own health. You can be in an emotionally intense, deeply intimate, lifelong relationship with someone, and that depth of feeling and importance will not be gutted if your mucous membranes never actually make contact with each other.

Pregnancy

While you're caught up in discussing STI prevention and kinky group play scenarios, it's easy to forget about the number one side effect of getting it on with someone of the opposite sex: pregnancy. Don't make the assumption that your partners are on the same page as you are. Make time to have straightforward conversations about what will happen if you, one of your partners, or one of your partner's partners gets pregnant unexpectedly. It is ultimately the pregnant person's decision, but that decision may potentially affect many different people and must be communicated accordingly.

If you are intending on getting pregnant, that must also be communicated to everyone involved. Your expectations for child-rearing may vary. You might envision cohabiting with the biological coparent of your child, or you may prefer to live separately and have many partners take part in child-rearing duties. Have these conversations with your partners earlier rather than later.

Sex Addiction

At the time of this writing, sex addiction, or hypersexual disorder, is still not listed in the *Diagnostic and Statistical Manual of Mental Disorders* (DSM). There has yet to be enough comprehensive studies and empirical evidence to sway the American Psychiatric Association, and there is still a clamor of contrary opinions. Compelling evidence suggests underlying biochemical causes of addictive or compulsory behavior surrounding sex—the same brain chemicals that can cause eating disorders as well as addictions to gambling and pornography.[10] But while many psychiatrists and patients insist that sexual addiction is a valid affliction, many others cry hogwash.

The term "addiction" is usually applied to scenarios wherein an exterior substance, such as drugs or alcohol, has created a chemical dependency in the brain. But applying the term "addiction" to behaviors is a little more wobbly. It doesn't help that the word itself is tossed around in a cavalier way. You can claim that you're addicted to buying Apple products, or that your husband is addicted to watching superhero movies.

In recent years, sex addiction has entered the public scope of awareness. Celebrities and public figures check into sex rehab after being caught in infidelity. Relationships undergo strain from one partner compulsively using pornography. And swingers and polyamorists, happily enjoying multiple sexual relationships, come under fire for having sexual needs that exceed the bounds of "normalcy." Is wanting lots of sex or masturbation normal? Or is that the sign of a crippling addiction in the making? Does being non-monogamous mean you're addicted to sex?

Critics of non-monogamy sometimes throw the sex addict label at swingers, couples in open relationships, and polyamorists, even though very few exhibit actual signs of it. While addiction is a serious issue, some skeptics have theorized that culturally we are too quick to pathologize behaviors that break outside of cultural norms.

Because there's no officially accepted definition to turn to, it is up to you to evaluate if your sexual behavior has become a problem. If you notice yourself having obsessive sexual thoughts that you can't escape, find yourself facing financial ruin because of paying for sex or pornography, notice that your need for sex is encroaching on your professional life and family life, or have an overall sense that you cannot control yourself or your sex life, then it may be time to find a professional or a therapy group.[11]

Sexy Pre-Sex Talk

If you're like me, talking about STI statistics and the merits of different forms of birth control triggers high-school-health-class yawns. Sex is supposed to be *fun*; why kill the mood?

This attitude is what prevents us from talking about sexual health and agreeing on safer sex practices with a potential partner before getting into bed with them. When you're in the middle of making out, caressing and grasping, sighing and moaning as clothes start to come off, no one wants to seductively whisper in their lover's ear, "Let's talk about STI prevention." Timing is everything.

The pre-sex talk should communicate information on your sexual health status and what kind of safer sex practices and birth control you are planning on using with this new partner, as well as what practices and prevention you employ with your other partners. (The new person should, by this point, be fully aware of how many other partners you have and know at least a little bit about who they are.) This conversation doesn't have to be dreaded or awkward, but it is best to bring it up to a new partner before sex is on the table at all. There is no one right way to do this. I once went on a first date with a man who told me about a major life overhaul, where he re-committed himself to eating healthy, staying active, speaking positively, and always having safe sex. It was the perfect segue to talk about what that specifically meant to him, far before sex was even a consideration between us. You might tell your date about this awesome book on polyamory that you're reading, and how fascinating and educational the chapter on sex is, and use that as a jumping-off point. Sometimes, a positive and direct approach also works well: "I *really* want to have sex with you, so let me tell you about X, Y, and Z."

Sexual Communication

Good sex incorporates physical pleasure, mental titillation, and verbal engagement. Talking about sex goes far beyond just knowing how to talk dirty (though that is an important skill). In a culture where it's still awkward to talk about sex at all, it's easy to get tongue-tied, even with someone you're close and intimate with. Pushing through this hesitation to talk about sex is the key to achieving a happy, healthy, and fulfilling sexual life.

This includes being able to discuss what you would or would not like when heading into a group sex situation. It includes being able to stop the action to check in with your partner to make sure she is doing all right and having a good time. It means drumming up the courage to share a long-held and slightly embarrassing sexual fantasy, and then exuberantly expressing to your partner afterward how amazing it felt to finally fulfill it. But most importantly, sexual communication involves being able to express or withhold consent.

"Consent" is a word that gets tossed around a lot, particularly in regard to wanted and unwanted sexual encounters. Seeking consent is not one gender's responsibility. Men, women, and people outside the gender binary are capable of having their consent violated. In any sexual situation, you have a dual responsibility: to make sure that your play partner is consciously and willingly consenting to the situation, and for you to enthusiastically and proactively communicate your own consent to your play partner. This does not have to be as dry as it sounds. (Giving a straight-up "Do you consent to this?" may be a mood-killer, but asking directly is necessary if your partner refuses to clearly communicate her feelings.) Instead, seeking consent can fit seamlessly into your ongoing conversation before, during, and after sex, such as:

I really want to kiss you right now. May I?
Do you want to keep going or do you want to stop for now?
Are you enjoying yourself?
And to give your consent:
I want to do X with you tonight. I can't stop thinking about it.
That feels incredible. Keep going!
I'm really happy that we got to do that.

As always, keep in mind that a person who is intoxicated may not be able to give consent or have the clarity of mind to ask for your consent. This doesn't mean that you and your partners need to be stone-cold sober at all times, but exercise caution, consideration, and good judgment, especially if engaging with someone you don't know very well.

Remember that consent can be withdrawn after it is initially given. This is very hard to do, especially for women, who have been taught to be nice and to not rock the boat by being a cock-tease. Sometimes it feels so much easier to do or say nothing—smiling politely and laughing it off when a stranger starts getting uncomfortably flirty, waiting for your partner to finish even though you're no longer enjoying the sex, or faking an orgasm in order to avoid hurting your partner's feelings. You might be afraid of the other person (or people) being annoyed with you, fearing that they'll get upset or angry and never want to have sex with you again. If this is the response you get, it's a clear sign that this person is not the right person for you to be having sex with anyway.

Consent and communication also apply to the sex itself, even after you've agreed to have it. We've all been in bed with someone who is attractive, intriguing, and exciting . . . but they're just not quite hitting the mark of what you like. Maybe they're going too fast, too rough, or not rough enough. Again, it can be difficult to speak up, because it feels so much easier to say nothing. In the past I've squirmed and wriggled, moving this way and that, attempting to position my body parts in such a way that whatever the other person was doing would start feeling good, or at least not feel painful. God forbid I should actually ask them to change what they're doing! That would just be rude . . .

Many of us have internalized this notion that if you're attracted to someone and getting high off of your shared chemistry, the sex will fall into place like it does in the movies. Close-up of locked eyes, swell of the background music, sprinkle in some passionate sighs, and cut to looking deliciously satisfied the next day. If only it were that easy. Again, it's tempting to fall victim to petty fears that the other person will find you demanding or picky or that you think they don't know what they're doing. Do yourself a favor and speak up earlier rather than later. Tell your partner if you like it faster, or a bit lower, or in a different position. Even better, find a time to let her watch you masturbate, so that she can really see which buttons to press for maximum enjoyment. I can guarantee that she will be much more excited seeing how much you're getting turned on, rather than being put off by your demands.

Chapter 6 Homework

Exercise #1

The next time you have sex (by yourself, one-on-one, or with multiple others), see if adding mindfulness enhances your enjoyment of the experience. Continually bring your focus back to your present sensory awareness. See how much detail you can pick up in the feeling of your partner's hand on your skin. Become aware of the rhythm of your own breath, and get curious about how it changes. When you notice distracted or negative thoughts arising, gently shift your attention back to the present and back to your senses. See if your ability to stay present enhances your enjoyment of the entire experience.

Exercise #2

It's time to get ready for that sexy pre-sex talk! Write down everything that needs to be communicated to a new sex partner so that you don't forget: your current sexual health and STI status, which methods you prefer to use for STI protection and contraception, and which methods you are using with your current partners. Some people choose to keep scanned copies of STI test results on their phone so they can be accessed at any time.

Remember that it's best to communicate these details before clothes start coming off. If you're feeling uncomfortable talking about these things, think about which things you might need in order to be more comfortable. A public space or a private space? Encouragement or support from your new partner? What are the things that you could do to make your partner feel more at ease talking about these things?

7 Land of Love-Craft: Crafting Your Relationships from the Ground Up

Everything is a mess.

The thought was playing on repeat in my mind. Over the course of about a year, my network of romantic partners devolved from a stable structure of supportive and loving relationships to total shambles. My girlfriend Emily, after much heartache and internal struggle, broke up with Jase, a mutual partner of ours, and also broke up with me in order to pursue a monogamous relationship. The tension and mistrust that had been brewing between Jase and my then-primary partner, Brad, erupted into multiple explosive confrontations. The feud left everyone hurting, nursing wounds that would take a very, very long time to close.

Years spent in steady and reliable polyamory had not prepared me for these failures. Despite running a podcast and blog on polyamory that was steadily growing in popularity, my own life was turning into an excellent example of what *not* to do. Even though I was coaching multiple couples and singles through the process of transitioning into non-monogamy, I was at a loss in managing my own relationships. In spite of quickly becoming a highly-sought "expert" on alternative love, I felt like I had no answers for my own problems. It seemed like the more I was learning about polyamory, the more mistakes I made in my relationships, and the more my control over the situation slipped through my fingers.

My turmoil was exacerbated by being caught in the cross fire of everyone else's opinions on the matter. Outside of personal stances on the people involved, everyone had strong and frequently conflicting viewpoints on what the very fundamentals of polyamory might be.

Brad was pro-hierarchy—*Polyamory means dedication to a primary partner. Everyone else comes second. All decisions have to be made with the commitment to the primary relationship in mind.* Jase, still smarting from feeling disempowered, was strictly egalitarian—*Polyamory means not letting any one person dictate what happens in other relationships. All partners get equal agency.* My partner Jake even started cracking jokes—*Polyamory means never having to say you're sorry! Polyamory means orgies on Tuesdays! Polyamory means responding to all text messages within forty-five seconds!*

And of course, there was a whole batch of concerned friends and family members throwing in their two cents as well, generally citing the situation as proof that non-monogamy is essentially impossible.

Everything is a mess.

Feeling like I was scraping the bottom of the sanity barrel, I decided to get out of town for a few days. I booked my accommodations, informed my partners of my plans, and hoofed it down to a beach city about an hour away. I ignored my social media and avoided text messages and calls. I didn't know exactly *why* I was making the temporary retreat; I just knew that I had to.

For a few days, the amount of silence, space, and stillness in my life drastically increased. After the rude shock of being deprived of sensory stimulation and entertainment had faded, after the constant buzz of judgments, opinions, and analyses had died down, after all the dust had settled, the resulting stillness allowed me to finally observe myself. I could witness the relationship I had with myself, with all of its strengths and flaws, as though I were witnessing a relationship between two people wholly outside of me. I could finally hear what it was I was saying to myself. On this self-facilitated retreat, I could hear loud and clear a huge realization: that I didn't even know what polyamory meant to *me.*

In the midst of listening to what each of my partners wanted and trying to keep all the plates spinning, I had completely lost sight of what it was *I* wanted. In the interest of maintaining the peace, I had forgotten that my desires existed. The forgetting was so complete that I could no longer remember what my needs, wants, and expectations had even been to begin with. I was determined to find my ground again.

Over the course of six consecutive hours, I wrote a document unlike anything I had ever written before. The piece flowed out of me as effortlessly as breathing. It began:

I hold these truths to be self-evident, that all human beings are created equal, that they are endowed by the nature of the cosmos with certain unalienable rights, that among these are life, liberty, love, and the pursuit of peace. That to secure these rights, relationships are instituted among human beings, deriving their form solely from the consent and desires of the participants. That whenever any form of relationship becomes destructive to these ends, it is the right of the participants to alter or abolish it, and to institute a new relationship or new form of relationship, laying its foundation on such principles and organizing itself in such form, as to them shall seem most likely to positively affect their safety, tranquility, and happiness.

Bearing in mind these truths, I, Dedeker Winston, in order to form a more whole human being, establish respect, insure interpersonal tranquility, provide for personal boundaries, promote the general welfare, and secure the blessings of life and of love, do ordain and establish this Constitution.

I wrote the Constitution of Dedeker Winston primarily to discover what I valued. I outlined specifically every responsibility to which I would hold myself in entering a romantic relationship, including maintaining honesty and transparency in communication, respecting the privacy of my partners, dedicating one-on-one time for each relationship, holding space for my partners to express thoughts and feelings—both positive and negative—and many, many more. I also detailed which rights I expected to be granted in my relationships, everything from being able to maintain autonomy over my personal choices to being able to travel with each partner.

The whole thing ended up being several pages long, and since I included an appropriate clause on allowing for amendments, it has undergone some revisions. Though the document was mainly for my own knowledge, I chose to share it with my partners. Some thought it was excellent, some took issue with certain parts, and the general consensus was that it was a little weird (breaking it down into regimented Articles and Sections was odd to everyone else, but logical, academic, left-brained yours truly absolutely loved it). Whether they loved it or hated it, the important thing is that it got each of my partners *talking* about what they also wanted and expected, and the things they were comfortable or not comfortable with. With my position clearly stated, it allowed for a foundation of collaboration, mutuality, and co-creation in each of my relationships.

That power to create is what has always excited me about polyamory. Growing up in Western culture, most of us are pretty familiar with the script for monogamous relationships. We know what it means to transition from saying "I'm dating this person" to "This person is my boyfriend/girlfriend." We know that the next step is living together, then marriage, then kids. And if we're unclear on any of that, we have plenty of places to turn to for advice.

Non-monogamous relationships don't have that same luxury. When I was growing up, no one taught me how to manage bringing multiple partners home to meet the family. There wasn't a book that covered what to do when one of your boyfriends becomes romantically interested in your other boyfriend. I never learned what it would be like to go on an amazing first date, and then come home and talk about it with my live-in partner. I went through a lot of trial and error before realizing that I had the power to create relationships that served me, my life, and my partners.

That is why it is so important to know who you are and what you want and need. Outside of the influence of your parents, your church, your workplace, or your group of friends, the possibilities for your life and your relationships are limitless. All those self-awareness inquiries in chapter 3 should set you on the path to a good foundation for personally crafting your relationships.

In this chapter, you'll learn more about the multitude of relationship structures most commonly seen in non-monogamous relationships. This chapter also digs into a controversial topic—whether or not "rules" are necessary for a successful non-monogamous relationship. If you are considering opening up a previously closed relationship, you and your partner may be feeling a strong urge to put several rules in place. This chapter will uncover what may be motivating you or your partner to suggest certain rules, and will help you carefully consider which rules or agreements may actually be needed. Hopefully, you'll come out of this chapter ready to cook up your own Constitution (or Operating Instructions or Relationship Contract or Ten Commandments or Mantra of Love or whatever official title gets your juices flowing).

The Romantic Alphabet

The two-person dyad has dominated our cultural views on romantic relationships. The United States Supreme Court decision in June of 2015 to nationally legalize same-sex marriage brought with it inherent controversy, but it also introduced a new topic of debate—if the definition of marriage could be changed to remove the limitation of only being between a man and a woman, could it also be changed to remove the limitation of only being between two people? There has been vocal opposition from both conservatives and liberals, and even within the non-monogamous community there is vast disagreement about the legal future of polyamory. There will be more information on that in chapter 11, but it's clear that defining, understanding, and legitimizing relationships that include more than two participants may become a public conversation in the future.

These multiple-person relationships take many forms, and no single format is inherently better or more successful than the others. Pay attention to which ones sound appealing, which ones scare you, or which ones excite you. You might find the autonomous nature of solo polyamory to be attractive, but you may also be enticed by exploring the dynamics of a triad. Remember that this is fluid, and that you can incorporate your favorite parts and aspects of different structures into a fancy new hybrid structure that works for you. When it comes to building your relationship frameworks, pulling a Dr. Frankenstein is encouraged (maniacal laughter optional).

Vee

A vee relationship looks exactly the way it sounds—like the letter V. One person in the "pivot" or "hinge" position is involved with two partners who are not romantically or sexually involved with each other. These two noninvolved metamours may be very close friends, or they may just be polite acquaintances. Some polyamorists are involved in more than just two dyad relationships that are not emotionally or sexually connected, expanding the V shape into more of a multi-pointed star or asterisk. Some people refer to this as their intimate network, or their polycule, or their web.

Triad

A triad is a three-person relationship in which all partners are romantically involved with one another. It may be one woman with two bisexual men, one man with two bisexual women, three people of the same sex, or a combination of three people who fall anywhere along the spectrum of gender identity. Some triads choose to live in the same home or raise children together. This nontraditional method of traditional homemaking often gets sensationalized airtime in the media, for better or worse.

A triad relationship rarely starts with all three people meeting one another at the same time. I've never personally witnessed a three-person first date where no one previously knew any of the others, but who knows what the future of alternative dating may bring? Two partners involved with the "hinge" partner of a vee may decide to become emotionally or sexually involved, making the relationship a triad. An already-established couple may form a triad by seeking a third person to become involved with both of them. This situation has become increasingly more common as sexual exploration and experimentation with non-monogamy slowly gains more visibility and acceptance. A heterosexual couple seeking a bisexual woman to become sexually or romantically involved with them has become so common an occurrence that there's even a derogatory name: "unicorn hunters." More on unicorns and unicorn hunters in chapter 8.

An individual in a triad relationship might still have outside partners, or even be involved in multiple triads at once! Some triads, however, choose to remain "closed" by practicing polyfidelity, where everyone agrees to avoid dating outside of the triad.

Quad

As the name implies, a quad is a four-person relationship. This can manifest in a variety of formats—two couples may become romantically involved cross-couple (kind of an X shape, if you're visualizing). Or one person from couple A may be involved with one person from couple B, forming an N shape. Polyamory can definitely change the way you look at the alphabet!

In the poly community, cross-couple quads have a reputation for being unstable. I would be reticent to label any structure as more unstable than any others. However, as you add more people to a joint relationship, you are also adding more concurrent sets of insecurities, preferences, and needs. Managing all of those things for multiple people is not impossible, but it can certainly be complicated.

For example, Anna and Kevin are a couple. They become involved with Theresa and David, with Anna entering a relationship with David and Kevin entering a relationship with Theresa. There now exist four romantic relationships that need to be cared for: Anna and Kevin, Theresa and David, Anna and David, and Kevin and Theresa. There are also the metamour relationships between Anna and Theresa and between David and Kevin. Even though these relationships may not be sexual or emotional, those connections still need to be fostered and kept healthy for the sake of harmony. There is also the relationship shared when all four people are together. That's a grand total of seven relationships! If any one of these connections suffers some kind of problem, it can and will send ripples through all of the others.

Solo Polyamory

There are a number of extant interpretations of solo polyamory, and few people agree on what the set definition might be. The solo polyamorist usually shies away from being considered part of a couple. Though she engages in multiple relationships, she may not feel a strong desire to cohabit with any one partner or take part in other activities that prioritize one particular romantic relationship over others. She is the one making all of the decisions considering her partners, but not necessarily allowing them to dictate or directly influence her choices. The solo polyamorist's relationships may be casual and transient, or they may be very deep, intimate, and loving. Or they may be a broad mix of many different levels of intimacy and emotional intensity.

Poly counselor and author Kathy Labriola distinguishes three distinct open relationship models:[1]

- *Primary/Secondary Model*—An established hierarchy wherein one relationship holds primary importance, and all other relationships are considered emotionally and logistically secondary.
- *Multiple Primary Model*—All partners are considered primary, or have the potential to become primary. Each partner is considered when making decisions about living arrangements, sexual connection, and time commitment.
- *Multiple Non-Primary Model*—All relationships are kept casual or less committed. An individual who is mainly committed to raising children, maintaining their career, or engaged in creative projects may choose to make that part of her life primary, while all relationships come second.

Solo polyamorists often employ either the Multiple Primary Model or the Multiple Non-Primary Model. In traditional romantic culture, the Multiple Non-Primary Model may sound similar to a person who we would say is "single" or "a free agent." Usually, this is a period between monogamous relationships, which may be spent dating or intentionally avoiding dating before the next long-term relationship comes along. For some people, solo polyamory does serve as a temporary phase between more intense relationships. If you value having one or many casual or non-intimate partners, you may live as a solo polyamorist until a more intimate or primary partner connection develops with one or more of your partners. Others choose to make solo polyamory a lifelong pursuit. Making the relationship with one's self the most important relationship is seen by some in the poly community as smart and independent, and by others as selfish and noncommittal.

Since the dissolution of my former relationship hierarchy, I have identified as a solo polyamorist. When Brad was no longer my primary partner, I knew that I wasn't prepared to go out and find another person to click into the primary slot. Nor was I interested in "upgrading" one of my other partners to position number one. Though my future may involve cohabiting and sharing finances with one or multiple partners, I've been content to handle these things solo for the time being. Many people come to polyamory seeking to establish one partner as the foundational relationship, and everyone else is just a bonus. After leaving what was formerly a foundational relationship, I realized that I myself could be the strong foundation upon which all of my relationships are built. My process of decision making has shifted from considering what would make my primary relationship the strongest and happiest to focusing on what would make myself and all of my relationships strong and happy. This approach may not ring true for everyone, but it has freed me to become my most authentic self.

Relationship Anarchy

The term "relationship anarchy" was first coined by queer feminist writer Andie Nordgren in a pamphlet she published in Sweden in 2006.[2] Because the movement is so new, people openly identifying as relationship anarchists are still relatively rare.

Relationship anarchy holds that all interpersonal relationships are important, not just those that are romantic. A relationship anarchist might engage in polyamory and have multiple, concurrent loving relationships, but may also avoid making special distinctions between relationships that are romantic, sexual, platonic, or familial. A relationship anarchist allows all relationships to self-govern, without external restrictions or expectations on what that relationship should be like. This includes eliminating distinctions between different categories of relationships, and instead allowing all relationships to take any form and have any level of commitment that the participants decide to have. A relationship with your best female friend would not be superseded by default by the relationship you have with your long-term, live-in boyfriend.

The relationship anarchy movement is still finding its feet, and it is sometimes misinterpreted as practicing a lack of commitment to anyone or anything. Relationship anarchists argue to the contrary, stating that love is abundant, and an individual should craft their commitments to fit each unique relationship. A strong foundation of self-awareness of one's relationship values is highly encouraged.

Labeling Love

We are used to describing our relationships to others with quick, easy labels. "This is my coworker." "This is my best friend." "This is my girlfriend." But when you have multiple romantic partners, what label do you use? Can you still call your partner "my boyfriend" if you've got multiple partners? Won't that confuse the heck out of everyone?

Labels are useful, but they can also force you to put your relationships in a box made by other people. Remember that labels should serve you, not the other way around. You will likely have to describe the shape of your relationship life to the skeptical or curious, but the labels you attach to your relationships should be your own choice. Poly people use a wide range of titles—boyfriends, girlfriends, partners, paramours, lovers, companions, soul mates, and more. If you are unsure if one of your partners is comfortable with a particular label, don't be afraid to ask.

Swinging

Swinging is the practice of having multiple sexual partners outside of a committed romantic relationship, sometimes within the context of a swinger's party or other such event. The swingers scene started gaining ground in the fifties and then picked up steam as a part of the free love movement of the sixties and seventies, as you'll recall from chapter 2.

There are many different approaches to swinging. Couples who swing tend to place priority on maintaining the primary romantic relationship, with all other partners kept to casual sexual relationships. Some couples only explore other partners at specific swinger's events and don't seek to maintain any relationships outside of these one-off encounters, but other couples choose to develop regular, ongoing friendships with play partners. People who identify as polyamorous may still partake in swinging experiences as well.

One of the arguable advantages of swinging is that a couple may choose to temporarily or permanently close their relationship if things are getting rocky. Because the outside relationships are not encouraged to have deep emotional connections, cutting them off for the sake of the primary relationship is less likely to result in feelings being irreparably hurt or hearts being broken.

Primary/Secondary Hierarchy

Just as most swingers choose one primary relationship to prioritize over all others, some people practicing polyamory do the same. The single primary relationship may be established as the most important, with all other partners being secondary or tertiary. These secondary/tertiary relationships can run the gamut from casual to emotionally intense and intimate.

A primary relationship can look many different ways. Your primary may be the person you decide to marry and have kids with, but still maintain outside emotional and sexual connections. He or she may be the person you choose to live with, though both of you may occasionally spend the night with others.

Hierarchal polyamory is clear in establishing certain relationships as being more important than others. For this reason, relationship hierarchy can be both a blessing and a curse. It is important to distinguish that hierarchy that arises in a manner that is prescribed, preset, or established is subtly different from a hierarchy that arises in a manner that is descriptive, organic, and flexible.

An organic, or descriptive, hierarchy organizes relationships based on the nature and circumstances of each relationship. Laura may have started dating Stan and Julia around the same time, but has found herself drawn to spending more of her time with Julia and later decides to move in with her. Laura might choose to *describe* her relationship with Julia as primary, considering their relationship has organically evolved to be deeper and more involved than her relationship with Stan.

But let's say, a year later, Julia has chosen to move away for a job opportunity, making her relationship with Laura long-distance. Stan has recently broken up with one of his partners, leaving him with more time for a relationship with Laura than he had before. If Laura and Stan develop a much deeper relationship and start spending most of their time together, then which relationship is primary? If we are looking at it through the lens of descriptive hierarchy, Stan could be described as primary. However, if Laura and Julia have decided to formally establish their relationship as the primary relationship, then Laura's relationship with Stan would have to be secondary, regardless of circumstances. Hierarchal polyamory is a subject of controversy in the non-monogamous community, for reasons discussed later on in chapter 8.

Hierarchy almost always comes into play if one relationship has a significantly longer history than others. This particular situation is faced by monogamous couples who are looking to transition into non-monogamy by opening up their relationship.

Open Sesame

Wanting to open up a previously closed relationship may be the very reason you are holding this book at this very moment. In my time spent coaching, I would estimate that three quarters of my clients are monogamous couples wanting to change their relationship structure to something non-monogamous, flexible, and "open." If this is you, compliment yourself for taking steps to educate yourself before embarking into what can be scary, unknown territory.

Changing the agreements and structure of your relationship is going to be both exciting and challenging, especially if you've been monogamous with your partner for a long time. You may have spent the entire relationship expecting that you would never have to closely examine the things that make you and your partner feel vulnerable, or that you would ever have to tease apart what specifically makes your relationship special and different from other potential romantic relationships.

This intense work is not wise to tackle if there are already fundamental problems in your existing relationship. If you and your partner have trouble communicating frequently, proactively, and transparently, then this may not be the right time or the right relationship for discovering non-monogamy. Polyamory cannot "fix" underlying issues, so commit yourself to uncovering the reasons why both of you want to take this step.

That being said, your relationship doesn't need to be perfect. You don't have to have a track record that's free of arguments. What you and your partner *do* need is a strong sense of self-efficacy. It might be helpful to review chapter 4 and take note of which attitudes and practices are present in yourself and in your partner and which ones might need a little work.

So where do you even begin? Both you and your partner probably have lots of hopes and fears for how your relationship will unfold after opening up. These hopes and fears may feel too vulnerable to share, but they are great material for learning more about yourself and your partner. These feelings and aspirations also set the starting point for your initial conversations about agreements, boundaries, or rules.

What's the Difference?

Whether you are opening up an existing relationship, or beginning to craft a network of many poly relationships, it is paramount to understand the functions of agreements, boundaries, and rules in your relationships. What distinguishes an agreement, a boundary, and a rule? All three can be used to structure a relationship in order to keep everyone happy and feeling safe. However, all three can also be implemented in a way that is destructive, inflexible, and manipulative. For the purposes of this chapter, here's what you need to know:

A *rule* is imposed by one person upon another person, or by one relationship upon another relationship. That doesn't mean that rules are always one-sided. Often couples may agree to impose the same rules upon each other. Rules also come with implicit or explicit consequences when they are broken.

A *boundary* is a limit or restriction that you place upon yourself. Some people refer to their boundaries as deal breakers or personal limits. If a person or situation crosses one of your boundaries, it is your responsibility to enforce the consequences upon yourself and no one else. This may involve physically stepping away from an uncomfortable situation or leaving an abusive relationship. Everyone has physical, emotional, and mental boundaries. However, not everyone is consistent in enforcing their own boundaries or in respecting the boundaries of others.

Lastly, an *agreement* is straightforward—something that two or more parties have agreed upon. In relationships, agreements may be clearly defined or may be informal and organic. Some people choose to formally write out their relationship agreements—*We agree to spend Friday nights together. We agree to text each other to say goodnight even when spending the night with someone else.* Others find an organic approach more freeing.

Rules Are Made to Be Broken

For being an incredibly adaptable species, human beings fear change, perhaps more than anything else. Remember how distressing the thought of switching schools or moving away to a different town was when you were a kid? Think of how many people you know (perhaps yourself included) who have stayed in a relationship far past the point of getting enjoyment out of it, solely from apprehension over changing the status quo.

Starting a new non-monogamous relationship or opening up an already existing relationship qualifies as big change for most people, which means a copious amount of terror comes with it. In the face of this distress, the knee-jerk reaction is to do everything possible to either soften the blow or to prevent the change entirely. In non-monogamous relationships, this usually manifests as a long list of rules. Believe it or not, it is possible to have a healthy, happy polyamorous relationship without creating any rules whatsoever.

This is the point where most people need to call a time out.

But everything will fall apart without rules! If my boyfriend can just run around and sleep with whoever he wants, why would he stay with me? How do I protect myself from the worst?

Most rules are put in place with the belief that without strict safeguards, the worst will happen. The "worst" could be your partner abandoning you for someone else or compromising your sexual health. Let's examine some common rules that a lot of people implement when first undertaking a polyamorous relationship.

- *It's okay for both of us to date other people, but I don't want to talk about it or hear about it.*

This is commonly known as a "Don't Ask, Don't Tell" policy. It falls under the category of controlling information in order to avoid jealousy (see chapter 6). The idea of hearing about your partner's awesome first date with someone new might turn your stomach into knots. The solution for many people is to not have to hear about it in the first place. Pulling an ostrich-head-in-the-sand act may prevent immediate uncomfortable feelings, but it completely shuts down lines of communication and obliterates an opportunity to generate more intimacy with your partner. Think of how good it feels to talk about a new crush or gush over an incredible date with your best friend. Getting to share that joy with a romantic partner, as well as receive it from them, can deepen your bond unlike anything else.

Intentionally keeping yourself in the dark can also have an unexpected side effect: your incredible, expansive, amazing brain will precision-target your deepest insecurities, and then imagine the worst possible scenario based on them. If you have no idea who your partner is dating, your brain will guarantee that it must be a supermodel who is taller, thinner, sexier, and richer than poor, short, chubby, awkward you.

Getting to learn about your partner's other partners might seem scary at first. I promise you, more information and more details will allow you an access point to feeling more in control, more comfortable, and more included. The fastest way to get the most information and inclusion is to actually meet your partner's other partners face-to-face. More on that in chapter 10.

- *If my primary partner doesn't approve of someone I'm dating, they can veto that partner. If I don't like someone my primary partner is dating, I can veto them as well.*

Notice that "primary" partner is distinguished in this one. This is because veto power often shows up in hierarchal primary/secondary arrangements. The idea is that if any secondary partner is perceived as a threat—in action, word, or persona—to the primary relationship, then that relationship can and should be terminated at the request of the primary partner.

The underlying fear here is that a new person could potentially steal away your primary partner or otherwise "come between" the two of you. The power to bring down the axe on any potential partner may offer a sense of security, but the price is high.

Take a moment to imagine if you had a veto agreement with your mother. You've both come to the consensus that your relationship as mother and daughter is important enough to deserve protection from anyone who might try to get between you. Now imagine how it would make you feel when your mother vetoes the brilliant, charming, attractive person that you are head over heels in love with. Your mom may feel more comfortable, but what state would your heart be in? Would your relationship with your mom get better or worse? Perhaps even more disquieting, what if you were on the receiving end of that? Would you enter into a relationship with a person who had such an agreement with their mother?

You can see how easily veto power can shift from being a source of security to a potential catalyst for disaster. If this is a rule you or one of your partners is considering, take some time to get to the bottom of your motivations. There are plenty of alternatives, covered later in this chapter, to help you feel more secure in your relationship that don't involve having to break any hearts.

- *You are not allowed to _____ with anyone else but me.*

You can fill in the blank with any number of things—spending the night, specific sexual positions or acts, going to a particular restaurant or venue, using a certain pet name, saying "I love you," going on trips, introductions to family members, etc. If your partner shares any of these special activities with someone else, the fear is that your relationship with him or her will then cease to be special and unique.

These kinds of restrictions have a common root—the prevention of intimacy. There is a tempting feeling of safety in thinking that you might have the power to prevent anyone else from getting as close to your partner as you are.

The specialness and closeness of every relationship is reflected in an infinite number of ways. The great thing is that every relationship has a specialness that cannot be replicated or replaced, because you yourself cannot be replicated or replaced. No one else has your smile. The way you philosophize on the nature of the universe has never been uttered by anyone else. You hold the monopoly on having a passionate love of impromptu dance parties coupled with a particularly extreme aversion to wearing clothes during said dance parties. The inherent uniqueness of *you* is what you bring to each relationship to make it special, and there is no one out there who can duplicate that (at least until human cloning becomes commonplace, but that can get covered in a later edition).

- *We can date other people, but only if we are dating the same person at the same time.*

Many couples theorize that no one will feel left out or jealous if a new partner becomes involved with both of them at the same time. This rule may also arise as the result of fears surrounding your partner having independent relationships. Mathematically, it seems to make sense. But human hearts are notorious for being really, *really* bad at math.

All relationships organically develop at a different rate and develop different needs along the way. You, your partner, and your potential new partner are all unique individuals, making each dyad within the prospective triad totally different. This makes it impossible to ensure that each relationship grows in exactly the same way, unless you and your partners have found a way to jack in to each other and enter hive-mind mode (again, depending on how the future unfolds, this may come up in a later edition).

This is often the basis for "unicorn hunter" relationships, covered in depth in chapter 8.

These are only a few of the possible rules and restrictions that may show up. Rules imposed by one partner upon another maintain a spirit of fearing change and discomfort, or paranoia that your partner will hurt you if he or she is not kept in line. The reality is that there is no rule that can ultimately prevent you from ever feeling hurt. No rule can force your partner to become inherently more considerate of you. The divorce rate in America is a glaring testament to the fact that even the ultimate legal rules established in standard wedding vows do not serve as a cure-all. This isn't the place to wax poetic about the fundamentally unpredictable nature of life and the illusion of security within a universe of impermanence, but at the end of the day, it is important to recognize that our efforts to tightly grasp a relationship or forcibly change the behavior of a particular partner are essentially fruitless.

That's beautifully logical, and it's also a huge bummer. Quasi-Buddhist syllogisms are great, but they are unlikely to help you feel much better when you're feeling twinges of jealousy while your partner is out on a date. So where is the good stuff? How do you avoid limiting your partner or your relationship while still maintaining a sense of stability, assuredness, and co-creation?

Boundaries

Boundaries are crucial to keep yourself safe and to maintain the integrity of your values. You may have physical boundaries that define who, when, where, and how another person is allowed access to your body or personal space. You may have emotional or mental boundaries that delineate the ways in which you feel safe being in intimate relationships. Most people have boundaries that extend beyond the sphere of romantic relationships: you may have boundaries regarding your choice of diet, your commitment to professionalism in your workplace, or your connection with your parents. Whatever your boundaries may be, the most important thing is to make sure that they are clearly defined to yourself and to others around you. Remember, a boundary can only be established by you, be applicable to you, and be enforced by you.

Take these three steps to make your boundaries clear.

1. Determine what behavior from others runs counter to your values.

These may be behaviors that you have already been tolerating. These may include dishonesty from your partner, seeing a sex partner make unsafe choices in their sex life, or invasions of your privacy.

2. Set a boundary that addresses that behavior.

Remember that boundaries are placed on yourself; they are not the yardstick to keep everyone else in line. There is no set formula for phrasing boundaries, but these examples may give you an idea:

I will not tolerate someone invading my privacy.
I cannot accept my partner lying or engaging in unethical behavior in her other relationships.
I will not permit anyone to call me names or use abusive language toward me.

3. Determine how your boundaries will be enforced.

If someone pushes one of your boundaries, and you do nothing about it, it becomes easier and easier to let other boundaries slip away as well. In order to avoid becoming a doormat, it is necessary to know what you will do to enforce your boundaries. Boundary enforcement doesn't always have to look scary and negative. If one of your partners is engaging in sexually risky activities or refusing to use protection with others, you may enforce your boundary by insisting on using boundaries for all of your own sexual encounters. Bear in mind that this shouldn't be a punishment of your partner, but rather a protection of yourself.

Boundary enforcement may just be a commitment to not letting something slide, making the choice to politely yet firmly speak up when someone crosses a line. Or it may mean removing yourself from a relationship with a person who is consistently inconsiderate of your boundaries.

Boundaries have a contradictory nature in that they are not flexible, yet they may change over time. You may enter a new relationship with a boundary against anyone reading your text messages or invading your privacy. Yet as time goes on and trust, honesty, and transparency become guiding values of the relationship, you may feel comfortable with your partner having access to your phone or email accounts for logistical reasons. As the circumstances of your life and relationships change, you may find that your boundaries shift. However, always be vigilant that your boundaries are changing of your own volition, not from pressure or coercion from someone else.

Agreeing on Agreements

The poly community enthusiastically embraces having set "agreements" in relationships instead of rules. You might argue that it's just semantics, and I've witnessed some strict relationship rules masquerading as agreements—*We **agree** that if you stay overnight with anyone else, your ass is grass.* However, there are important philosophical distinctions that separate the spirit of an agreement from that of a rule or boundary.

One of Aesop's fables, *The Oak and the Reeds*, illuminates it best.

> *A very large oak was uprooted by the wind and thrown across a stream. It fell among some reeds, which it thus addressed: "I wonder how you, who are so light and weak, are not entirely crushed by these strong winds."*
>
> *They replied, "You fight and contend with the wind, and consequently you are destroyed; while we on the contrary bend before the least breath of air, and therefore remain unbroken, and escape."*[3]

Like the reeds, agreements can bend and shift with circumstances, with personal growth, and in response to mistakes. Rules, like the oak, get broken in the face of resistance. As you talk with your partners about the kind of agreements you want to uphold in your relationship, be mindful of the some of the most important qualities of a successful agreement:

It considers all people involved.

A good relationship agreement takes into account the needs and humanity of every partner. A rule such as "No spending the night with anyone else" lays the groundwork for preventing another person from getting what they need. Your girlfriend's new partner probably doesn't want to steal her away from you, but getting to occasionally share a bed with her may be important to him for sustaining a happy, connected relationship.

We can take sexual health as an example. Non-monogamous sexual practices are a charged topic, and mindfulness and consideration is paramount in this arena. An agreement about sex that considers every partner might look like this:

I agree to clearly communicate sexual history, STI status, and safe sex practices with all partners. If there is any foreseen or current change in any of these things, it will be discussed with each of my partners.

Under this agreement, if you and one of your partners want to start having unprotected sex, it would be discussed with all of your other partners, since it affects their sexual health as well. This does not necessarily mean that you're seeking permission from all of your other partners, but it puts the power in their hands to communicate their concerns and make further negotiations to protect their own sexual health.

Negotiation is welcomed.

You are a living, breathing human being. (I assume. The list of science-fiction future topics for the next edition just keeps getting longer and longer.) Your relationships are organically growing, evolving entities. Your agreements should be the same. No one likes feeling like they are under the thumb of the law. Holding the space for flexibility and negotiation gives breath and vitality to each of your relationships.

Suppose this is one of your agreements:

I agree to maintain complete transparency of information and total honesty in communication with each of my partners.

Honesty with a lack of omissions upholds an environment of trust and good communication, so this is a great foundational agreement. However, let's say that Rebecca's partner Owen opens up to her one night about some childhood trauma that is affecting his sex life. When Rebecca's other partner, Helen, asks her how her night with Owen went, how much should she communicate? After all, she agreed to not omit anything!

It may seem like an obvious decency to protect the privacy of others, but I've seen this violated numerous times in poly relationships. I was once in a primary relationship where my partner demanded to be able to read all of my text message conversations with other partners, without allowing me to communicate to them that he would be privy to these private conversations. The relationship did not last long.

Being an open book is an admirable quality, and it is better to share more information with your partners rather than less. However, in this situation, Owen may feel uncomfortable with that personal information being revealed to Helen by default. In the spirit of negotiation, Rebecca might choose to alter her agreement to this:

I agree to maintain complete transparency of information and total honesty in communication within the realm of respecting the privacy of each of my partners.

Or, she may add a new agreement:

I agree to seek consent before sharing any information about a partner that may be of a personally revealing or private nature.

Some people are very private, and some people couldn't care less what other people know about them. It will be up to Rebecca to have conversations with Owen (and with Helen) about what kind of information can or should be shared.

Trust, not fear, is the guiding light.

We all have fears of being alone, of being abandoned, of being unwanted and unloved. Some of us are ruled by these fears more than others, but they are universal. It can be so tempting to build a proverbial fence around someone you love, hoping against hope to prevent ever losing them. All of the negative rules discussed earlier in the chapter mask a desperate plea: *Please don't leave me alone!*

No sugarcoating it—trusting your partner's love is freaking scary. Even in a monogamous context, handing your heart over to someone is one of the most vulnerable things you can do in your lifetime. Despite this, human beings keep allowing themselves to fall in love. Repeated trial and error has shown us that the benefits outweigh the risks.

Create your relationship agreements from a place of trusting that your partners love you and have your happiness in mind, rather than the fear that your partners are going to hurt you. Give yourself and your partners the gift of forwarding your trust, even if you don't feel it 100 percent. It will be worth it.

Minimalism

"*You know you have reached perfection of design not when you have nothing more to add, but when you have nothing more to take away.***"** —Antoine de Saint-Exupéry

Take the time to write out a list of boundaries, a collection of guidelines, or a manifesto for yourself before creating something similar with one or multiple partners. Figuring out where you stand and what you expect of yourself will produce something much more detailed and comprehensive. After all, you know (or are getting to learn) all of your strengths, weaknesses, and insecurities. All of your ins and outs. When it's time to come to the table with one of your partners in establishing agreements for your relationship, that comprehensive self-knowledge will allow you to do something that may seem counterintuitive at this point: simplify.

Yeah, the person who wrote a ten-page Constitution for herself is telling you to simplify. Just bear with me.

Once you've compiled something representative of your values and agreements, whether they are your personal guidelines or created with your partners, try to find the common thread. See if you can discover a single guiding principle that would sum it all up. Can you write that principle in one sentence? In one word?

Finding the fundamental essence of your agreements doesn't mean you have to scrap all the specifics, but it allows you to cut to the heart of what is most important to you and to your partners. It's unlikely you'll be able to come up with agreements for all contingencies. Situations that you completely did not expect can and will happen. Having your single motto can act as a solid baseline when circumstances throw you for a loop. A few of my favorites that I've seen:

- Honesty over harmony.
- No surprises.
- Be flexible.
- Treat others *better* than you want to be treated.
- Don't be a dick.
- Trust over fear.

Chapter 7 Homework

Exercise #1

Before coming up with something poetic or refined, it's time to get messy. Just start writing. Write a list of the things you definitely want from your relationships and what you definitely *don't* want. Use profanity. Or crayons. Don't be afraid to be selfish, or to completely ignore all of the advice in this chapter. Let your vulnerable, emotional self take the wheel for a little while. You probably won't show this version to anyone else, but it's an important first step.

Exercise #2

Take a look at your vision for your ideal romantic life (from the homework for chapter 3). Now consider what kind of person you would have to be in order to deserve your ideal love life. What responsibilities would you have toward your partners? What personal qualities would you need? What kind of agreements would make your ideal love life feel safe for everyone involved?

8 The Good, the Bad, and the In-Between

For a long while, I was the excited flag-waver for hierarchical poly- amory. After all, being polyamorous had made me outrageously happy. I was over the moon for my primary partner, Brad, whom I was moving in with. I was fast falling in love with my new secondary partner, Jase. And I was exploring my first relationship with a woman with my partner Emily. Emily had been with Jase for years and had started dating Brad shortly before dating me. We all had other partners, but it was our little poly quad that became infamous in our circle of friends. We rolled into parties, taking delight in quelling our friends' shocked reactions with our polished poly rhetoric. To most of the people we met, we were ambassadors of open-mindedness, sex positivity, compersion, and abundant love. It wasn't long before we got pretty full of ourselves. Brad and I started discussing poly rights activism, and Jase began crafting plans of creating pro-poly content to generate awareness—books, podcasts, workshops, etc. These were the first baby steps toward the creation of Multiamory.com. All of us, and myself most of all, were convinced that we had it all figured out.

When it all fell apart, I was at a loss. Before finding the quad, I had already spent years of trial and error, making all the newbie mistakes. I thought that I had already done my time. These relationships had been proof to me that, if you go about it the right way, it could all turn out perfectly. Now that assurance was quickly crumbling, and I didn't know what to do. After seeing the highs of a polyamorous life, I was loath to witness the deep, dark lows.

The times of breakups and meltdowns weren't only dark, but confusing. I had never had to puzzle so much over what relationships actually meant to me and what the right course of action was. This confusion has been echoed many times over in the stories that I hear from my clients (and may perhaps be the reason why I have a coaching business at all). People in alternative relationships don't yet have the benefit of a culture chock-full of role models, media, books, and movies demonstrating how healthy non-monogamous relationships should go (though that is changing). There are a lot of people with a lot of questions, and not enough established answers.

Even within the polyamorous community, there is debate over how much advice and guidance one can give. After all, one of the primary "selling points" of nontraditional relationships is that you get to craft your relationships to look however you want them to. Is it anyone's right to tell someone else "You're doing it wrong"? Wouldn't that just be perpetuating the same cycle of judgment, discrimination, and stigma shown toward alternative relationships and sexualities?

I'm happy to say that I rediscovered that initial happiness and joy, that sense of belonging, security, and trust, and an even deeper appreciation of my relationships. I once again enjoy multiple strong relationships with dedicated and loving partners. But that rediscovery came with the understanding that polyamory, like any other form of human relationship, is far from perfect. I learned that it was okay to carry the flag, but I didn't have to wave it in my friends' faces. And I also discovered that between the brilliant joys and troubling sorrows is the puzzling middle ground: controversial relationship structures and common predicaments that still cause heated debate within the poly community. To this day, for every relationship quandary I think I've figured out, a client or a friend comes along with a whole new one. As time goes on, I come closer to accepting that when it comes to relationships, there are very few hard and fast rules, there are virtually no absolutes, and everything is relative.

In this chapter, you'll get a glimpse of each facet: the good, the bad, the in-between. The benefits discussed in this chapter may not even hold a candle to the great joy that you discover, and you may never sink to the depths of any of the lows mentioned. (At least, this is my greatest wish for you.) But understand that the more unique people you add to your life, the more unique relationship situations will be sure to follow, for better or worse.

The Good Stuff

So you've waded your way through self-awareness inquiries, communication workshops, personal development, finding quality partners, negotiating agreements, figuring out your boundaries, taming your twinges of jealousy, navigating scheduling conflicts, gracefully diverting horrified reactions to your lifestyle, and explaining your relationships to your parents for the fiftieth time. Welcome to polyamory! It's easy to think, "Why did I get into this in the first place?"

It takes work to keep all of the plates spinning, but many have discovered that the joy and satisfaction found on the other side is worth far more than the cost of admission. If non-monogamy resonates with you, there are few words to describe the fulfillment to be found when your inner desires are congruous with your outer life. Outside of this holistic sense of actualization, there is a whole world of good stuff to sink into.

Abundance

There's much discussion about "enough." We worry if we are rich enough, smart enough, pretty enough. We worry if we are receiving enough pay, enough recognition, enough attention, enough sex. We ourselves want to be enough, to our parents, to our bosses, to our partners. And how many times has the average poly person been asked, "You don't think one partner is enough?"

In monogamous relationships, we are expected to be everything, and we expect our partners to be everything. Your spouse or significant other needs to be your romance-novel beloved, your best friend, your kinky play partner, your coparent, your therapist, your caretaker, your policeman, your personal trainer, your support group facilitator, and maybe even your parent at times. It's a lot of expectation to put on one person, but that's just what the job description is. Finding someone who is enough to fill all of those roles simultaneously is a tall order, and hats off to those who can not only fill that order, but sustain it 'til death do you part.

Proponents of polyamory often point to the benefit of having multiple people fit multiple needs and taking this pressure off of a single partner and off of yourself. And indeed, when the pressure is off, it creates space to discover what each person can bring to the table even if they can't bring *everything* to the table. The problem is that the things that we need from other human beings are not cut-and-dried. We aren't able to cherry-pick partners and mark off our checklist of needs in an attempt at finally getting "enough"—*Let's see, I've got Sam for good sex, Andre to father my children, Lisa for cuddling on Tuesday nights, and Josh for binge-watching anime. Needs fulfilled!*

The harsh truth is that you are not enough. Your partner is not enough. Multiple partners are not enough. Your parents are not enough. Your friends are not enough. But if recognizing this is disturbing to you, it's because of the way you are looking at the concept of "enough." It is said best by the poet Nirmala:

the truth catches up with me
I am not enough
never have been
never will be
what relief to admit this finite container
can never contain infinity
what joy to find infinity needs no container[1]

Human needs are infinite, and our capacity to be fulfilled is infinite. In the same way that you are incapable of getting enough breath at one time or enough food at one time to sustain you for the rest of your life, it is impossible to get enough of anything from any of your relationships that will keep you satisfied forever and in all circumstances. In certain periods of your life, you may need good, exploratory sex not just from one relationship, but all of them. In the same period, you may feel happier with lots of alone time and not need a lot of focused attention from others. But at other times, sex may become less of a priority, and you may find yourself needing lots of attention and focus from your partners. You may go through phases of enjoying many first dates and creating new connections, and other phases of focusing solely on your existing relationships. But at any given time, your relationships give you the flexibility to seek whatever it is you need, and in abundance as well. There is not just an abundance of affection, attention, and love, but an abundant potential to find fulfillment even as your needs for those things change. For this reason, long-distance relationships are particularly suited to polyamory. Being out of close physical proximity with a loved one may not be ideal. But if both of you have the freedom to meet your needs for attention, affection, and sex with a variety of people, the cost and stress of maintaining a long-distance relationship is drastically reduced.

The best non-monogamous relationships not only allow for multiple needs to be met with multiple relationships, but are flexible enough to provide for a shifting landscape of needs. In the personal Constitution I wrote for myself (see chapter 7), I outlined the things that I knew that I needed in all of my relationships—things such as honesty, kindness, open communication, and one-on-one time. These base needs do change slightly, but for most of my time being poly they have been basically the same. As long as I am getting those things, whatever else my partners bring to the relationship is a uniquely wonderful bonus.

"There is a moment I remember from each of my monogamous relationships, it's a sickening, sucking-hole-in-the-gut feeling of grief, when you realize that you just are not enough for the person you're with. In a monogamous relationship, that's the moment that breaks hearts. You were supposed to be this person's 'everything' and yet here's a need or desire you either can't or won't fill, and where do you go from there, how do you reconcile that?

The best part of being polyamorous, for me, is knowing I don't have to. I feel like it would be rather selfish of me to expect anyone I love to be wholly satisfied with just me, to expect someone to compromise deep feelings of need or desire for my benefit, just like it would be selfish of someone else to ask me to compromise personal boundaries I have to meet the needs that they have. With polyamory, I get to experience the happiness that comes from my partner being completely satisfied as opposed to their taking what they can get.**"** —Lila

"For me in particular, [my partners'] diversity means that for anything I need to talk about, there is at least one of them, usually two, who can offer a perspective that will greatly enrich my own understanding, and help me reach a resolution in my own feelings and thoughts. They all collectively and individually supplement my perception of reality, expanding the comparatively narrow framework from which I alone would tackle life. I'm a better person because of them.**"** —Mia

Don't forget that not only do you reap the benefits of love from multiple partners, but you also have the potential to receive an abundance of support and connection from your entire network of metamours and friends.

"I love the relationship that I have with husband's girlfriend, she's my best friend. The three of us hang out together when she comes to visit, we have even gone on trips together. We plan gifts for my husband, we sew and craft together, she's helped me try to get jobs. One night the three of us were hanging out in a hotel hot tub, talking about our 'cheat codes': things that help us calm down in stressful situations, or how we would prefer those close to us to react when we're upset. We plan on eventually living together, and it's my hope that she will be a major part of my eventual children's lives.**"** —Bria

"So many things about [polyamory] are the best. The built-in support system we have. Having partners with really different interests who expand my horizons and fulfill different parts of me. Conspiring to surprise a partner or metamour with the perfect birthday/Christmas/whatever gift. Double the hugs when I come home from work. The joy I get from seeing my partners happy and growing into themselves with the help of their *partners. More people to help eat all the things I want to bake but couldn't possibly finish on my own . . . I could go on and on, really.* **"** —Rebecca

Agency

Having personal agency is traditionally defined as having a sense of control over one's life and actions. But it's important to avoid confusing a person who seeks agency with a person who seeks to control or dominate. It may be more appropriate to look to the philosophical definition of agency: a living entity's capacity to act in any given environment.[2]

All good relationships require the participants to have a sense of agency. We jokingly make references to who "wears the pants" in a given relationship, but effective romantic relationships require a collaboration and synthesis of multiple individuals' needs. In order to have your needs met, you must have the agency to act and to express yourself: to ask your partner for the things you need, to lend your voice in decision making, to be an active participant in your relationships. No one wants to be silenced, disregarded, or disempowered. Even in 24/7 Dom/sub relationships, it's still necessary for the submissive to have a say in the structure of the relationship and be able to voice his consent.

The hallmark of agency is not only the capacity to act, but the ability to do so in any given environment. As time passes and circumstances change, as you and your partners encounter breakups, finding new relationships, switching jobs, moving to different cities, and any other number of curveballs life throws at you, how do you create relationships that are sustainable? Many turn to polyamory because it allows them to craft relationships that fit their lives and their circumstances, rather than forcing their lives to fit the shape of a traditional relationship. People whose lives require that most of their time and energy be dedicated to work or children, or people who cannot be in close physical proximity to their partners, often turn to polyamory as a flexible solution.

The polyamorous are also particularly adept at maintaining agency when a relationship is not working: when someone's needs are not getting met, when interest or attraction has faded, or when the participants have simply grown in different directions. While this usually warrants a breakup or divorce in monogamous circles, polyamory allows for flexibility. If sexual attraction has waned between two people, but the relationship is still a source of love and care, the people involved are free to transition the expectations of their relationship to something different without having to abandon it entirely. De-escalating will be covered later in this chapter. It's an appealing option if circumstances are no longer making it easy to conduct a relationship, though it does require careful negotiation:

"*The most recent development in my relationship with [my partner] is this: She's moving to a very far-away city. I'm thrilled for her! I'm also thrilled to be more autonomous and move our relationship into more relationship anarchy style and less of a hierarchical style of relationship. It feels to me that we are de-escalating our relationship in a way, and I feel fine with this. She, however, wants to keep rigid labels around us being in a primary relationship. To me, we have primary aspects to our relationship; however, I don't feel the need to structure and limit things by way of labeling. This is an ongoing conversation.***"** —Paige

---

New Relationship Energy

Polyamory also allows for an abundance of NRE. New Relationship Energy, or NRE, is the term that poly folk use to refer to the hormones and emotions that people experience when developing a new relationship. These chemical changes are very strong for the first few months and can last for over a year as they slowly revert back to normal levels. They are the classic "falling in love" feelings: butterflies, ecstasy, hearts fluttering and eyes moony. If you're in poly relationships, it's likely that you'll experience NRE many times as you pursue new relationships. Bonus!

However, people in poly relationships can attest that NRE is a double-edged sword. While it feels fantastic, it can also make it easy to neglect existing relationships. If you are in the throes of NRE, the best tactic is just to be aware of it. Know that you're riding a chemical cocktail, and enjoy it as much as possible, but don't make any major life decisions. If you have a partner experiencing NRE in another relationship, understand that the fever will pass, and don't feel bad about asking for reassurance, time, or affection if you need it.

Compersion

The term *compersion* is the darling of the polyamory movement. Seriously, go talk to any poly person who has read all the usual reading material, and they will drop the word no later than five minutes into the conversation. Not only is it a word uniquely coined by polys themselves (the Kerista community, from chapter 2), but it describes a feeling that is largely unrecognized: feeling positive emotions about a partner being with someone else. Some call it the opposite of jealousy, though it is possible to experience both jealousy and compersion at the same time.

People who believe that polyamory is a more enlightened way of living are particularly fond of talking about compersion, because it offers up proof of enlightenment: *I am so magnanimous and open-minded that I have risen above the petty jealousies of the plebeians.* I used to think that compersion was essentially just tolerating your partners having other partners without flying into a jealous rage. I thought it sounded nice, but it was probably nothing more than a pro-poly term designed for sound bites. I operated this way for a number of years until I experienced compersion myself for the first time.

One day I watched one of my partners grab his girlfriend and plant an affectionate kiss on her cheek. I didn't know his girlfriend very well at this point, and I still felt twinges of insecurity and jealousy when my partner was heading out on a date with her. But seeing the huge smile break across her face suddenly set fireworks off inside of me. I couldn't resist grinning, myself, and I was caught off guard when I realized that witnessing the scene had generated only positive emotions. Feeling true compersion for the first time was both confusing and thrilling. For the rest of the day, I was floating.

For some people, compersion comes on with that same explosive quality every time. For others, it's a quiet realization. You may be unable to contain your thrill over a partner going on a first date, or it may not be until a year into your partner's other relationship that you recognize that subtle inner warmth and appreciation of your partner's happiness. It may feel like the best thing in the universe, or it may feel strange, new, and confusing.

As mentioned above, experiencing compersion does not necessarily make you immune to jealousy. You may feel nothing but compersion for one partner, and still feel insecure about another partner. You can even feel the two simultaneously about the same relationship. I've felt twinges of jealousy about a partner getting to go have a fun day at the theme park with his new girl-friend while I'm stuck at home with a cold, but still felt the glow of compersion knowing that it was exactly the kind of break that both he and his girlfriend needed from their high-pressure jobs.

"*I am happy that my husband has a lover with whom I have no physical con-nection; I am glad he has another person to love. What I most enjoy are the times I see my beloveds being appreciated and loved by other people. My stance is, 'Yes, aren't they great! I'm glad you see them as being great too.'* **"** —Jen

The Bad

I'm hesitant to label this section as "The Bad." There are few true absolutes in this universe, few things that are objectively good or bad. From our limited human perspective, it is impossible to know what is positive or negative in the long run, but knowing that doesn't prevent us from chasing after the good and running away from the bad (remember the amoebae from chapter 6). But it's incorrect to paint an image of polyamorous relationships that is all sweetness and warm fuzzy feelings. The "bad" in any type of relationship cannot be avoided; you can't have the yang without the yin, the up without the down, the peak without the valley.

Breakups

No one likes to talk about breakups. Breakups contradict the things we think we know about so-called true love: that it's eternal, invincible, and capable of conquering all obstacles. And that isn't necessarily untrue. Love can reach those depths and aspire to those heights. However, breakups and divorces often have nothing to do with love itself fading or disappearing entirely. Often, the reason why the end of a relationship hurts is because the people separating still love each other very much.

There are good reasons and bad reasons to end a relationship, but I won't give you an outlined list. Deal breakers are individually defined and depend on context. I have no personal dietary restrictions and care little about the diet a partner chooses, but this may be a source of fundamental incompatibil-ity in some relationships. I've had many relationships end because my partner decided that polyamory was not his cup of tea. That's a deal breaker for me and many other poly folk, but some people choose to create mono/poly relationship structures instead (more on that later in the chapter).

If a relationship has taken on unhealthy dynamics, it's likely that your friends and family members will know it's time to bounce much sooner than you will. However, only you can know when it's the right time to make the decision to leave a relationship, and only you can take action on that decision. It will almost always be a difficult call to make, especially if you still love the person and have no desire to hurt them outright. If you are struggling to know whether it's time to stay or go, I recommend asking yourself a single question:

If nothing changed about my partner from here on out, would I still want to be in the relationship?

This hypothetical question helps to highlight your true feelings about the relationship, and acts as a gateway to other important questions: Are you counting on your partner changing some fundamental aspect of herself? Do you see a future of having the same argument five, ten, or twenty years from now? Do you see the current rough patch as a solvable problem or as a recurring pattern? What part of your behavior and your partner's behavior would have to adjust in order to sustain the relationship? Finding these answers is an important step on the road to clarity about your relationship.

People think that ending a relationship is easier for someone with multiple partners. On the surface this makes sense: if you have multiple boyfriends and girlfriends to comfort you, surely it doesn't matter as much if you lose one of them! But many poly folk will attest that the pain of a breakup is just as acute as a monogamous relationship. It's the same way that having multiple children or multiple friends doesn't inure you to the pain of losing one of them.

However, there is one priceless benefit I have found to having other partners around while you are in the midst of a relationship ending. If you are in an unhealthy relationship and you know in your heart that it's time to leave, there may be a number of obstacles keeping you from biting the bullet. If you are living with your partner or sharing finances, you may be worried about finding a place to live, or fretting over how you will meet your financial obligations when you suddenly have a single income. You may be concerned about feeling a whole slew of negative emotions: loneliness, embarrassment, heartbreak, depression. Faced with the specter of instability and negativity, it's easy to choose to stick it out in a situation that is not working. An unhappy relationship isn't easy, but it feels like less work than finding a new apartment and separating your possessions. Staying with an incompatible partner hurts, but it seems less painful than facing the sting of loss, shame, and disruptive change.

Having a multiple-partner support network will not protect you from this pain, but it can help remove these obstacles. Having multiple partners who love you can vanquish those ridiculous gremlins that pop up when things are looking dark: *Where will I stay? I'm going to be so lonely. No one will love me again.* Your self-doubts and fears of being unlovable, unattractive, and undesirable are harder to keep alive when you are surrounded by an abundance of love, affection, and sex. This helps you get a little bit closer to the realization that everything is going to be okay, which frees you to face a breakup with a little more inner peace and fortitude.

When it's time to break up, whether it's initiated by you or by your partner, remember that it's not an outright failure. The length of time a relationship lasts is not an accurate indicator of whether it was successful or not. Even if the relationship you are leaving was unhappy, abusive, and destructive, it doesn't do any good to beat yourself up over time lost or mistakes made. Ideally, you will face future relationships with a little more wisdom, a little more clarity, and a better idea of how to be your best possible self and inspire your partners to be the same.

Never lose perspective on how a painful ending may give rise to new beginnings and new joy. In the words of Ralph Waldo Emerson:

> *Though thou loved her as thyself,*
> *As a self of purer clay,*
> *Tho' her parting dims the day,*
> *Stealing grace from all alive,*
> *Heartily know,*
> *When half-gods go,*
> *The gods arrive.*[3]

Transitioning and De-escalating

Non-monogamy forces you to be brutally honest when you are facing the end of a relationship. One can no longer hide behind the usual maxims: *I found someone else. I want to focus on my career. I think we should see other people. It's not you; it's me.*

It's harder to give these excuses to someone who knows that you are still perfectly happy to carry on relationships with your other partners. Instead, you have to address the actual root of the disconnect: *I'm no longer attracted to you. I want to focus on other relationships. I don't think we are compatible. It's not me; it's you.* Truthful? Yes. Easy? Heck no.

However, cutting straight to the heart of the problem grants an opportunity to examine if, rather than end the relationship, it's better to transition the relationship to something that better serves the people and circumstances involved. In a traditional monogamous context, a breakup or divorce is a kind of transition: from husband and wife to coparents, from boyfriend and girlfriend to just friends (or mortal enemies, in some cases). In a polyamorous context, these transitions are more fluid, often because relationship labels are more fluid as well. If you and your partner go from seeing each other every day to seeing each other every few months with weekly Skype calls in between after one of you moves out of town, what are you now? Did you make the leap to "just friends" territory? Or are you still lovers? If there's no longer a sexual attraction in your relationship, but you are still passionately in love and happy to share a home and raise a family together, does that mean the relationship has taken a step backward?

I encourage you to approach relationship transitions with a sense of flexibility and of possibility. If you and your partner would be happier if the relationship were de-escalated (perhaps seeing each other less frequently or reducing frequency of contact), it isn't a failure. As relationships evolve, it is never taking a step backward. Instead, it's just another step on the path to organically finding a relationship that is in the best possible shape for the people involved in it.

Abuse

Abuse is a dark manifestation of a loving relationship gone way, way wrong. The unfortunate thing is that warning signs of an abusive personality rarely show up early in the relationship. If someone started pushing you around, physically or verbally, on the first date, it's unlikely it would lead to a second date! Abusive relationships develop over time, with small breaches of boundaries here and there. Franklin Veaux and Eve Rickert, authors of *More Than Two*, refer to this as "concession creep"—when you concede to a partner's unreasonable demands or needs little by little, until you've found yourself without a leg to stand on. By the time the victim realizes that she is in an abusive relationship, usually the behavior has already been going on for a long time.

Abuse presents itself in different ways, but all of them involve attempts at control. Physical abuse includes unwanted physical contact, inflicted by one partner on the other. Things like slapping, kicking, punching, biting, throwing objects, grabbing hair, or coercive or forced sex. Verbal and emotional abuse may include general or targeted unkind behavior, such as calling the victim names or attacking his self-esteem, yelling and screaming, making threats to leave the relationship or otherwise cause emotional harm, delivering ultimatums, threatening suicide, or making the victim feel guilty for enforcing his boundaries or asking for his needs to be fulfilled. There is also financial abuse, wherein one partner keeps tight control over finances, keeping close watch over the other partner's spending, and disallowing their partner from being able to access bank accounts or maintain any kind of financial independence.[4]

Using the term "abuser" is charged. No one is born into this world as an evil abuser. Often, people who abuse are charismatic, loving, affectionate, and gregarious. Emotional abusers are particularly hard to spot, even when they are in the midst of doling out abuse. This is because an abuser will often believe that he himself is the victim. When the abuser's partner makes choices about her life that he does not agree with, he may accuse his partner of being hurtful, of attacking him, or of being the true abuser in the situation. He will claim that his partner's actions justify the abuser's use of name-calling, threats, or guilt. As the victim internalizes her partner's accusations over time, she may begin to believe the bad names and the accusations. Victims of emotional abuse often suffer guilt that paralyzes them, preventing their standing up for themselves and leaving the dysfunctional relationship.

Polyamorous relationships are not immune to abuse, and a poly context can set the stage for uniquely nasty manifestations of emotional abuse. Many poly folk carry a sense of guilt over being poly (aptly referred to as "poly guilt"). If you hold the belief that polyamory is something that your partner is just tolerating or is just letting you get away with, it's a slippery slope to seeing your partner's every outburst, insult, or bad behavior as justified. After all, you are the "bad" one by putting your partner through polyamory! Poly guilt creates the fertile ground for any number of abusive behaviors: forcing you to change or cancel established plans with other partners for nonemergency reasons, insulting or bad-mouthing your partners, dictating how often you are allowed to see other partners, controlling the level of contact or intimacy you are allowed to have with other partners, coercing you into having romantic or sexual relationships with your metamours, and many others.

Lastly, one of the most heinous tactics of emotional abuse is gas-lighting. Gas-lighting got its name from the 1938 play *Gas Light* by Patrick Hamilton, wherein a husband mentally manipulates his wife into thinking that she is insane, including lowering the gas-lighting of the house but insisting that she is imagining any change in the lighting. An emotionally abusive individual will get the victim to question his perception and feelings by controlling the narrative of what is actually going on in the relationship. Poly relationships are particularly prone to this because there is usually a lot of discussion about feelings. It is easy for one partner to insist that the other partner's feelings are incorrect. *You're not supposed to be jealous of me texting my girlfriend. It's not right for you to want to go on a date with someone else when I'm here feeling lonely.*

When one partner in the relationship claims to be the only one who has a grip on reality, be on the lookout for trouble ahead. It is natural to have arguments and to discover conflicting viewpoints. However, in healthy relationships, all partners can acknowledge that there are, in fact, different perspectives. Even though your partner may totally disagree with your perception of an event, she should be able to acknowledge that viewpoints alternate to her own are possible. Within all of your relationships, there has to be space for competing narratives and alternate realities to exist (not in a sci-fi way, though we'll see where we end up in a few centuries). An emotionally abusive partner will be convinced that she knows what's best, knows what's really going on, and knows your own feelings better than you do.

Abuse may be difficult to spot early on, but knowing how to recognize it is imperative in being able to escape it. If you are not sure whether or not you are in an abusive relationship, that may be the first warning sign. Educate yourself on patterns of abuse and reach out to a trusted friend or professional who is poly-friendly. Recognizing abuse lets you break above the surface of hurt, low self-esteem, and self-doubt and escape a harmful situation before it gets worse.

The In-between

I wanted to call this chapter "The Good, The Bad, and the Ugly" because it's one of my favorite films of all time, but it's not fair to attach the "Ugly" label to the relationship situations in this section. These particular relationship structures are common, but controversial. It is difficult to point a finger at any particular non-monogamous relationship configuration and proclaim it wrong. On one side, supporters will claim, "There's no one right way to do polyamory! Everyone is different!" And the other side will respond with the adage coined by Miss Poly Manners on the *Poly Weekly* podcast: "There's no one right way to do polyamory . . . but there are plenty of wrong ways!"

What is wrong and right is relative to each individual. If you find yourself in a relationship format that echoes the ones discussed below, take a moment to check and make sure it is truly making you happy. Beyond that, also ask yourself if it is making not only you and your partners happy, but your partners' other partners as well. If it's all good in the 'hood, you're probably on the right track and needn't worry about criticism from others. But if you're finding that not everyone is exactly thrilled, it's time to double check the pros and cons of being in this situation.

Unicorn Hunting

Imagine a happy triad relationship between three people. The triad is closed, meaning they only have sexual and romantic feelings for one another. They make a lovely little clan: sharing breakfast in the morning, spending lazy afternoons cuddling on the couch with video games, and playful, steamy threesomes at night. They get all the stability of an established, committed relationship, with the added bonus of variety and kinky sex! What's not to love?

Many couples seeking to spice up their relationship by dabbling in non-monogamy find the image of the happy triad enticing. Some couples in particular are drawn to the idea of having a regular threesome partner who isn't a random stranger. However, the desire to explore a triad relationship of whatever intensity often clashes with the fear of having to change the couple's relationship. Even worse, what if that new person tries to steal away just one half of the couple?

This fear of change leads the couple to seek a third person to shoehorn into their relationship, but only under a set of strict conditions: the new partner must be equally attracted to both members of the couple and develop equally intimate relationships with both. She can only engage when both halves of the couple are present; no pairing up for one-on-one dates, cuddles, or sex. She cannot do anything that may be perceived as "getting between" the two original partners. She can come over for group cuddles or threesomes, and she may even move in with the couple and be expected to share housework and child-rearing duties, but she must disappear if any family members, coworkers, or friends drop by. She cannot pursue any partners outside of the triad. Lastly, she has to conform to all of these conditions without protest. If she doesn't, she can take a hike. What's not to love?

The couple seeking the blissful triad arrangement may think they are being up-front on their dating profile by stating, "We are looking for a closed triad." In reality, it is false advertising, as they usually fail to include all of the unspoken expectations behind it. Any couple can be guilty of this, but the most common culprits are heterosexual couples seeking a bisexual woman to complement their relationship. As you can imagine, bisexual women willing to enter a relationship under these conditions are few and far between, hence the term "unicorn." (Would the male counterpart be a "pegasus"?) However, couples who are on a desperate hunt to find a unicorn are annoyingly commonplace in online dating site and poly meet-ups.

Many couples who come to me for coaching hear about unicorn hunting and are quick to reassure, "Oh, we would never do that. We would treat our third well." This misses the point. Very few unicorn hunters are seeking to find someone to abuse. But you can still treat someone like a princess while not allowing her power to make decisions in the relationship, which is more like owning a pet than having a relationship.

It's this mentality that sabotages the triad from the start. Instead of seeking a triangular relationship, where each leg of the triangle has a voice, most unicorn hunters are seeking a T-shaped relationship. The primary couple establish themselves as the most important relationship, and from the get-go it's "us" vs. "you." It is "our" girlfriend. Sadly, this dynamic almost always leads to hurt feelings and confusion for all parties involved. The unicorn may leave the relationship, frustrated at having no rights and alienated by being mistrusted from the start, and the unicorn hunters end up equally frustrated that can't seem to find someone who can seamlessly click into the pre-made slot they have crafted.

So what's the good side of all of this? As a matter of fact, there are far more unicorns out there than meet the eye. There are plenty of people who love the idea of a happy triad, and even some who are drawn to the idea of dating an established couple. However, as some self-proclaimed unicorns say, the bait that unicorn hunters lay is not the most appealing.

If you are seeking a happy triad, whether you are a mythological creature or a wandering hunter, there are some important guidelines to keep in mind. A healthy triad relationship aims to be a triangle rather than a T. This means that there needs to be space for each leg of the triangle to grow into individual relationships. Each relationship in the triad may not be totally equal, but they do need to have one-on-one time in order to grow and be able to stand on their own. The healthiest triads I have ever witnessed have also formed organically: rather than a couple seeking a third, one person started dating two people separately who also happened to start dating each other afterward.

There is one litmus test that I give to all couples who are thinking about finding a unicorn or otherwise adding a third. If you can envision yourself going on a first date with your third *alone*, or envision your partner going on a first date with your third *alone*, then you are likely off to a good start. If that very image gives you pause, and you'll only feel comfortable going on that first date as a couple, you may not yet be ready to add a third.

Balancing the Scales

A heterosexual couple decides to open up their relationship. They have a discussion about agreements and boundaries. They praise each other and make each other feel secure. They even help each other create online dating profiles. Everyone feels positive and excited.

Within moments of creating her profile, the female half of the couple has already received five or six messages from interested parties. In his inbox? Crickets. But that's okay! These things take time. He continues to send out hopeful messages over the next few weeks, as she starts scheduling first dates. Her first dates come and go, leading to second dates. He still can't get anyone to maintain an online conversation without ghosting after a while.

As she explores exciting new relationships, he tries not to get depressed. The women he is interested in online don't even give him the courtesy of a "no," and the women he meets in person are shocked and disgusted once they learn he is in an open relationship. As he watches his partner head out the front door to spend the night with her new squeeze, he has the begrudging thought that an open relationship was a horrible idea.

This story has been echoed countless times. These gender dynamics seem to plague newly non-monogamous heterosexual couples in particular, but the fear of an unfair or unequal relationship dynamic can affect anyone. Some people try to insure against relationship imbalance by making rules ahead of time. *You can only go on a date if I've got a date lined up. You can only spend the night elsewhere if I've got someone else to sleep with too.*

Discrepancies in the number of partners or frequencies of dates are not the only things that can make relationships feel unequal. Often there is conflict if two people have vastly different styles of dating. One person may prefer to have several casual partners or may seek out casual sex, while the other prefers to seek only a few partners and develop deeper connections. Conflict arises when the romantic relationship–focused partner can't understand why his partner wants so much sex, and the casual connection–focused partner can't understand why her partner is so emotionally wrapped up in his relationships. Again, some people turn to rules to solve the problem: *we agree to only seek out one-night stands, no getting the heart involved.* Or *we agree to only pursue romantic relationships, no casual sex whatsoever.*

But things hardly ever play out so evenly. You may not get much enjoyment out of casual sex, but your partner is over the moon by getting to play with a wide variety of people and doesn't have the time or energy to dedicate to a more time-consuming relationship. There will be times of feast and of famine. Sometimes you'll find yourself bummed out and cranky because you can't lock down a date and you're having arguments in all of your other relationships. Other times, you'll find yourself on top of the world, drunk on NRE, and full to bursting with love and affection. Even when things are good, it can be easy to see the grass as greener. I've been heading out to my third date of the week while burning with envy that all my partners already have long-term, bonded partners. And I've been enjoying many intimately connected, meaningful relationships and still felt envious when one of my partners is going on a lot of exciting first dates. Our feelings are rarely if ever logical.

So why is this an in-between? Forcing equilibrium to happen in a relationship is disastrous, and yet the actual experience of equilibrium can be invaluable. I've coached numerous people who struggled to come to terms with their partner's other emotionally intense relationships. But when they themselves fell in love and wound up in an emotionally intense relationship of their own, it served as the key "a-ha!" moment that made everything easier. Often, the best way to understand your partner's experience is to step into their shoes and try on that experience for yourself.

Should you aim for equilibrium in your relationships? Yes, but not if it requires you or your partner to restrict or inorganically force a change into your relationship behavior. Seek an organic equilibrium based on mutual understanding and trust, rather than on needing external circumstances to look equal at all times.

Mono/Poly

The mono/poly hybrid relationship is a unique beast. This structure occurs when one partner in a couple chooses to remain monogamous, while the other one is openly non-monogamous. These relationships may form at the onset of a connection. A poly person may find themselves falling head over heels for a monogamous-leaning person or vice versa. Or a mono/poly relationship may come about when a formerly monogamous couple decides to open up the relationship at the request of one person.

You can probably guess that this is an arrangement particularly prone to conflict. In practice, relationships between a monogamist and a polyamorist end up with one partner having to accept a disproportionate level of compromise. The couple may choose to practice monogamy, which generally results in unstable dynamics. The poly person may unhappily restrain their desires and inwardly hope that their partner will come around to polyamory in time, or the monogamous partner will feel paranoid that their formerly poly partner will someday ask to open the relationship, will cheat, or will leave the relationship to seek other partners. Or the couple may choose to practice one-sided polyamory, but this dynamic may not produce healthy results either. The mono partner may be holding out hope that this poly "phase" will eventually pass. The poly partner may worry about causing harm or sparking jealousy in her mono partner, which impels her to restrain herself in communication and in seeking new partners.

It's common sense that two people with vastly different life goals may not be compatible in a relationship. If a church-going nine-to-fiver (who wants to settle down in the suburbs with three kids and a dog) falls in love with an atheist freelance artist (who wants to spend the next five years backpacking across the globe), it is unlikely that a committed relationship would make either of them happy in the long run. Even if these two people loved each other very much, the relationship would not be able to work without huge compromise on both sides. This would involve compromising career goals, spiritual beliefs, and life plans. It isn't impossible to compromise on these things, but it is tricky to find a middle ground where neither side feels like they have given up too much of themselves.

Mono/poly relationships are the same. It is difficult to find a compromise between two vastly different relationship approaches that will not leave one or both sides feeling resentful. In spite of this, people still power through, trying to make an incompatible relationship work, mostly due to the belief that if their love is strong enough, they can handle anything. What many people entering incompatible relationships fail to realize is that love is powerful, amazing, and life-changing, but at the end of the day, *love is not enough.* Love may create a deep bond and inspire beautiful intimacy between two people, but if those two people are fundamentally at cross-purposes, then love is not enough to make it all work.

That being said, there is a sprinkling of mono/poly success stories. The most successful examples I have seen have been relationships wherein one partner can no longer have sex (due to illness, loss of sex drive, or other reasons), finding stability and relief when the other partner is allowed to seek sexual fulfillment elsewhere without having to sacrifice the established relationship. But even these success stories are few and far between.

Effective mono/poly relationships require both partners to strive for near-unconditional love for each other, which is difficult for any human being. There has to be a baseline of full acceptance; each partner must be willing to accept each other exactly as they are, without any hidden desires to change the other person. And both have to be willing to endure considerable growing pains as each person tries on individual compromises. It *is* possible to have a mono/poly relationship, but bear in mind that it requires willingness on both sides to endure lengthy negotiation, processing, and discomfort.

The One Penis Policy

The One Penis Policy, or OPP as it's usually called, involves an agreement wherein a man can have one or more female partners, but those female partners are not allowed to have male partners. Sometimes this also shows up in mono/poly couples, where the monogamous-leaning man is okay with his female partner being open and polyamorous, but only with other women. Only one penis allowed, hence the name.

The flip side of OPP is a One Vagina Policy, where a woman would be allowed multiple male partners, but those male partners could not engage romantically or sexually with other women. There are no formal statistics on the frequency of OVP relationships versus OPP relationships, but anecdotal evidence within the poly community suggests that OPP relationships are far more common.

It's important to note that there is a difference between single-gender dating naturally occurring in one's relationship versus it being laid down as a strict policy or rule within the agreements of the relationship. Many queer people take part in these kinds of relationships, not because it's part of the relationship agreements, but just because they are not particularly interested in pursuing individuals of a certain sex. There are also people in BDSM Dom/sub relationships, where restricting access to the sub's partners or specific sexual experiences is a part of the power play, but this restriction may be lifted when not in the realm of sexual play.

In these two instances, it's *descriptive* OPP at play. There is no formal policy or rule; the circumstances are just such that only one man is engaged in the relationship at that given time. And it makes sense. If a person genuinely has no interest in pursuing men as it is, then there should be no need for a policy to be laid down restricting it.

When OPP is established from the outset, then things get tricky. Many people justify prescribed OPP as a "baby step" on the way to a fully open polyamorous relationship. If the man is too threatened by the notion of his female partner getting involved with other men, the theory is that his experience of her dating women might be a gentler, easier-to-swallow step on the road to an open relationship. Many people espouse the practice of moving forward at the rate of the slowest person, not forcing anyone to rush into something they are uncomfortable with. This thinking is understandable, but requires two important factors be in place in order to be successful:

1. The woman must be bisexual. That may seem obvious, but I've witnessed a number of men just assuming that their female partners will have a healthy interest in women that is equally as intense and fulfilling as their interest in men.
2. It eventually transitions to an equal-opportunity open relationship once the man feels safe.

Unfortunately, number two seems to be the sticking point for many OPP relationships. The idea of other male partners may never feel as "safe" as female partners do. The couple may find themselves waiting for a comfort with other men that never actually arrives.

So why is this the case? Feminists will cry havoc and claim that these men are just trying to hunt down a threesome or that these men don't think that romantic relationships between women are "real" relationships. As you'll recall from chapter 6, there is no denying the widely held view that bisexual female relationships are transitory, experimental, "girlish fun." There have been many cases of men in OPP relationships who get an uncomfortable wake-up call when they realize that their female partner's new relationship actually has a life of its own, with needs for emotional support, communication, and one-on-one time. This can be a particularly challenging realization if his partner's relationship with a woman is autonomous, and he does not have any kind of romantic or sexual access to her girlfriend. What's more, these policies rarely take into consideration the possibility of the female half of the couple dating a transgender person. This of course begs the question: is it the ownership of male genitalia or is it a masculine appearance and identity that would be more threatening to her cisgender male partner?

It's dangerous to paint people with a broad brush. There are few open-minded men out there who consciously think that female-female relationships are fake or disingenuous. It's also unlikely that these men are nothing but insecure control freaks crippled by their own sense of competition with other males. The common justifications for single-gender non-monogamy are presented much more logically.

You may think that your partner dating someone of the opposite sex from you is safer because, after all, they offer something that you can't. There's no direct competition! It's true: if your partner dates someone of the opposite sex from you, it does offer a unique dating experience, the opportunity to explore new realms of sexual exploration, and it fulfills different needs.

On the flip side, you may feel tempted to require that your partner only date someone of the *same* sex as you. After all, what if your partner discovers something so amazing, so interesting, so unique in the opposite sex . . . and there's literally no way you can compete with body parts that you don't even have?

The irony is that whenever your partner dates someone else, regardless of their gender, it opens up the possibility for finding something unique, exploratory, amazing, and fulfilling. The benefits of having multiple partners extend beyond what genitals happen to be attached to those partners. If the only thing holding back you and your partner from a fully open relationship is insecurity surrounding a particular gender, then face it head-on. Talk openly with your partner about what makes either of you feel uncomfortable or threatened. Brainstorm ideas on how to change your thinking or how you can help each other feel more reassured and stable in your relationship. And if you or your partner absolutely insists on using single-gender dating as a baby step, make sure that you establish a time frame when you will check in again and take the plunge into equal-opportunity dating.

Primary/Secondary Hierarchy

I covered hierarchy briefly in chapter 7, but now it's time to really dig into why relationship hierarchy has become so controversial in the poly community. If you are brand-new to non-monogamy, and especially if you are looking to open up a currently closed relationship, hierarchy may appear quite logical. Your boyfriend or husband or wife or life partner clicks in to the special role of "primary." Your primary's needs and desires come first, and you know that your primary will put your needs first as well. This hierarchy allows your primary relationship to enjoy the benefits of standard monogamous relationships —stability, security, intimacy, planning for the future, life entwinement—while also enjoying sexual and romantic variety.

Primary/secondary hierarchy is still popular today, but its roots come from the early days of the modern polyamory movement. By and large, it's an old-school model. Many of the polyamorists of the eighties and nineties borrowed rules and agreements that worked for the swingers of the sixties and seventies. Swingers (then and now) usually format their relationships in a hierarchy: one person is the primary (or anchor) partner, and that relationship is emotionally monogamous. All other relationships are only for sexual variety or to spice things up for the primary relationship. At that time, most polyamorists extended this to their relationship models as well. Relationships outside of the anchor relationship were considered by default to be "secondary." While these secondary relationships might grow into intimate and meaningful romantic connections, it was still important to make sure everyone knew their place. That's just the way it was done. And that's exactly what I thought when I first stepped into the world of polyamory.

My Experience with Hierarchy

I wholeheartedly adopted the primary/secondary model from day one. As I was learning about non-monogamy, I internalized the values of generous love, of being noncompetitive, of embracing sexual freedom, and I preached these things to others. When it came to confronting my own jealousy issues, I was short-sighted. Logically, I understood all the usual advice about jealousy in poly-amory—that's it's just an emotion that passes, that it doesn't mean my partner doesn't love me or is going to abandon me, yadda yadda yadda. But my emotional side hadn't caught up with the logic. I still felt that inner knife twist when I knew my partner was away with someone else.

That is, until I discovered that I could establish a hierarchy in my relationships. I realized that if I knew that I was the queen bee, that I was the only person my partner truly loved, and that everyone else was less important to him than me . . . poof! Jealousy gone! I enjoyed a number of non-monogamous relationships this way, feeling secure in the knowledge that I was receiving plenty of love with no real threats to my position. As long as my partner's other relationships were all kept casual or primarily sexual, I had no jealousies whatsoever.

When I began my relationship with Brad, it took about six months before I learned that he had another partner, and that he was in love with her as well. It was the first time I had ever been in this scenario, where love and affection, not just sex, was being given to someone other than me. It sent me into a tail-spin of inner conflict. I had read so many books on polyamory. I knew that in theory, everyone should be free to love as many people as they wanted. That there shouldn't be any competition. But I couldn't stand the thought that the person I was in love with might be giving equal or, even worse, *more* love to someone else. How could I feel secure in that situation, knowing that I might not be priority number one?

Driven by panic and insecurity, I fought to become priority number one. I asked Brad to spend holidays with me months in advance, fearing that if I didn't secure the date, he would give it to someone else. I made myself as available as possible, shifting my schedule and canceling any engagement that conflicted with the times that he told me he was free to spend time with me. I was tender and saintly as he told me about fights he had with his other partner about scheduling conflicts and her jealousy issues. I prided myself on being "the good child"—never making any complaints even when I was upset, never pushing my jealousy on him even when I was seething with it, never contradicting him even when I disagreed. When Brad and I finally established each other as primary partners, I breathed a sigh of relief. Finally, security! At last, I could relax and not give a hoot what he did in his other relationships, because I was number one.

The problem was that security and relaxation never really arrived. Now that I had made it to the top of the mountain, I had to defend my position as king of the hill. Any activity that Brad engaged in with other partners that seemed "primary-ish" (such as making travel plans, introducing partners to his family, engaging in new sexual explorations, or even accompanying a partner to a doctor's appointment) would instantly turn my stomach. The problem with being granted primary status was that I knew it would be just as easy for Brad to take it away from me and give it to someone else. The thing that I thought was my only source of security could vanish at any moment, and I lived under constant fear of the ax coming down.

My thinking started to change as my secondary relationships developed and matured into deep, emotional connections. Remember the section on finding equilibrium? When I also had partners outside of Brad that I wanted to travel with and introduce to my family, it became clearer to me that it truly was possible to love and prioritize multiple people, without anyone missing out. Brad and I, both drunk on the joy of being in love with each other and with others, talked about how much we enjoyed being primary to each other, but that we also didn't want our other partners to be labeled or treated as secondary. We agreed that we would never establish any kind of veto rule or restrict each other from developing intimacy with others. Brad began connecting to his metamours, we began exploring the new dynamic of dating and falling in love with another couple, and I furiously meditated and read self-help books to try to confront my feelings of threat from Brad's other partner.

I wish this was the happy ending I could leave you with. But the dynamic that Brad and I chose to establish for our relationship would not be sustainable. We didn't realize that it is impossible to have a quality romantic relationship with a new partner, where you can give yourself deeply and vulnerably and receive the same from them, but still maintain that at the end of the day, someone else will always come first, will always be more important, will always hold the throne as the primary partner.

After Brad and I moved in together, things began to turn sour. We were excellent at running a household together, but it was our feelings toward each other's partners that began to grow tense. I was frustrated that moving in with Brad still had not inured me to jealousy and the fear that he might form a deeper bond with his other partners. Under the surface, he started becoming resentful of the growing depth of my relationship with Jase, though he didn't express his feelings to me until much, much later. He had encouraged my dates and sleepovers with Jase, and he had even spoken positively about witnessing us being affectionate and having sex with each other during group play sessions. I felt grateful for Brad's support of my other relationships, but as my relationship with Jase began to take on a life of its own, that support started to withdraw. Our fights got worse; he started calling me names, hitting things, throwing objects across the room. I cried and cajoled and pleaded and argued, but over and over again I made the choice to stay with him.

One day, Brad snooped through my email accounts, social media accounts, and text messages. He read every conversation I'd had with my mother about my jealousy issues, flirtatious texts with my girlfriend Emily, conversations between Jase and me about our sex life, including sexy images we had taken of each other and anonymously shared with others. Brad flew into a rage of hurt and spite, and from that point on, things were irrevocably different in our relationship.

When I felt insecure and jealous, I sought to fix it through becoming the primary partner. In Brad's insecurity and jealousy, he did the same, reinstating a strict hierarchy with a vengeance. While all of my other relationships got his blessing and support, it was my relationship with Jase that got crushed under the steamroll of the established hierarchy. Brad knew he could not veto Jase, so he demanded that I spend less and less time with him. He forbade me to wear jewelry that Jase had given me. It got to the point where I even avoided saying his name. "Every time you mention him," Brad told me one day, "I think 'Fuck Jase' in my head." When I objected, Brad called into question my commitment to the relationship, and whether or not I was living up to his standards of what it meant to be a primary partner. When I quarreled with him, he suggested that maybe he hadn't chosen the right primary. Perhaps one of his other partners was actually supposed to be his true primary. It was the nightmare I had feared from the very beginning.

I pulled away from Jase, seeing him for a bare minimum amount of time in order to keep a ghost of a relationship alive. Over and over again, in the midst of nights spent in tears and my hair starting to turn gray from the stress, I chose to stay with Brad. What else could I do? He was my primary, and I was his. The hierarchy that I had fought for for so long, the primary partner status that I had held up as the hallmark of security and commitment, became the leverage that was used against me. Despite the hierarchy no longer serving me whatsoever, I couldn't bring myself to abandon it.

I still don't know what impelled me to stay in the relationship with Brad as long as I did. Perhaps it was that certitude in hierarchy. The belief that once I had earned the top rank, that meant unquestioning sacrifice for the person I had committed to. Thinking that boundless love meant having no personal boundaries. Feeling so sure that if I could just show how much I was willing to give, that I was willing to hurt others who I love and to hurt myself, that it would make everything better. But with everything that I sacrificed, neither Brad nor I succeeded in feeling better. I knew that Brad wanted me to end the relationship with Jase, but he openly admitted that even taking that step wouldn't guarantee the end of his anger and insecurity.

The end of my relationship with Brad came with the full weight of all the pain that we had intentionally and unintentionally inflicted upon each other. My other partners consoled me through each agonizing stage of grief as I tried to pull myself together and understand why things had gone wrong. I was angry at myself for tolerating the relationship as long as I had, and simultaneously devastated at the loss of someone I loved.

It was the unending kindness, understanding, support, and love of my partners, metamours, and community that got me through to the other side. It took months for the fog of pain to lift, but when it did, I saw the great treasure trove of wisdom to be found. For so long, both Brad and I had sought security in the format of the relationship, rather than in each other and within ourselves. Our obsession with maintaining the hierarchy created an inflexibility that turned the positive aspects of love, intimacy, connection, and exploration with our other partners into threatening forces of chaos that sought to destroy the fragile house we had built for ourselves. In seeking to preserve our primary relationship, we had sucked the joy out of our other relationships.

So what wisdom did I take away for myself? It may surprise you to know that this experience did not lead the pendulum to swing the other way. I didn't start preaching strict egalitarianism in relationships, nor did I become jaded and cynical. I'm happy to report that I didn't swear off having intense, emotionally entwined relationships for fear of being hurt again. (Though that fear certainly crossed my mind more than once.) Rather, my thinking about relationship importance shifted from primary/secondary to focusing on priority, flexibility, and fluidity.

Priority Versus Primary

Sadly, my story is not unique. You'll find many tragic stories of secondary relationships suffering or ending entirely for the sake of preserving a primary relationship. The primary partner may have felt threatened by the secondary partner, or the people in the primary relationship may have established strict rules that disempowered all secondary relationships. On the other hand, many people insist that relationships need to be clearly defined for the benefit and security of the participants. From that standpoint, the common assumption is that if someone has a problem being secondary, they should either find their own primary partner or avoid getting involved to begin with. This practice works well for swinging, because the emphasis is on fun, casual sexual exploration, rather than on developing heart-based relationships.

It's undeniable that every human being has a set of priorities. For some, financial stability is a priority, leading them to put most of their energy into saving money and seeking out smart investments. For others, career advancement is the top priority, inspiring the drive to chase advancement in the workplace and to develop a strong resume. In the same way, different relationships take priority for different people. Some people put their kids before anything else, others focus on romantic relationships, and still others concentrate on maintaining a healthy relationship with their best friend of twenty years. It is natural for us to prioritize certain people over others in certain situations. When deciding which school to put your kids in, you may seek the opinions of your coparent and perhaps your friends, but you may not reach out to your parents or to your boss at work, even though those relationships are still important to you. When faced with a tough decision about switching careers, you may consult with your family or your best friend, but probably not with the person you just went on a first date with.

Unless you are a staunch relationship anarchist, it's unlikely that you'll ever be able to keep all of your relationships truly equal, even if you are actively trying to avoid a strict hierarchy. Life circumstances, changes caused by personal growth, and the unpredictability of human emotions will cause your relationships to shift in importance and intensity, regardless of your best efforts to keep everyone in a particular place in your heart.

If you have been happily married for ten years and you are now looking to try out polyamory, of course I'm not going to tell you that you need to knock your spouse down a peg and no longer make that relationship a priority. But I will say that there needs to be a commitment to making room for other relationships to be a priority as well. We make room for shared priorities in many areas of life. If you are totally jazzed about signing up with a personal trainer, it would be strange if your boss came to you and said, "Hey, best of luck with your trainer! But please don't do more than one session per week. I don't want you to get so involved with working out that your job is no longer a priority for you." If you and your spouse were getting ready to have a baby, it's unlikely your spouse would come to you and say, "I'm really excited we're doing this together. But please make sure that our relationship always comes first, okay? I don't want this baby trying to get between us and break us up." Yet this is the attitude many people take when faced with the prospect of adding new partners.

Human hearts are tender, squishy things. If your interest is in finding multiple love relationships, establishing strict hierarchy is the equivalent of shoving other people's hearts into cookie cutter shapes, and putting up barbed wire fences keeping them at bay. In order to love, our hearts need softness, flexibility, and careful handling (and the occasional padded room). They require a fluidity of feelings, emotions, and relationships that mimics the constant inflow and outflow of your blood. The boundaries you place on your own heart need the gentle yet clear stance of a line drawn in the sand, not the outright aggression of a barricaded fortress. Whichever type of relationship structure you gravitate toward, if human hearts are on the line, you must find the guiding lights of flexibility, fluidity, and above all, compassion.

Chapter 8 Homework

Exercise #1

Bring to mind a breakup from the past. What are the valuable things you gained from experiencing the end of the relationship? What lessons did you learn about yourself and how you want to conduct your relationships moving forward? If things got nasty during the breakup, what could be done to avoid the same thing happening in the future?

Exercise #2

Many of these "In-between" relationship structures come about due to one person or both people in the relationship wanting to feel important and not wanting to feel threatened. What are ways that you can make someone feel special outside of imposing these relationship formats? How do you reassure someone of their importance outside of granting them primary status? If your partner is threatened by a particular gender, how can you calm your partner's fears without swearing off dating that gender?

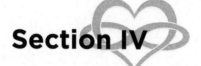

Section IV

Out of the Classroom, Into the World

9   Say Good-bye to the Closet

You are being led by Satan.

That was the text message my partner Jase's girlfriend received from a family member not long after the two of them started dating. When this family member cyberstalked Jase's Internet presence and discovered his open polyamorous identity, her reaction was less than pleasant. Jase was disturbed by the sudden realization that this might happen again with future partners. "I used to always be the guy that every parent loved," he lamented. "Now am I always going to be the guy that no one wants their daughter to date?"

I had experienced a similar feeling when a new partner told me that he had told his parents that I was a professional author currently writing a book on psychology. I laughed it off because it made me sound impressively smart, but afterward I was hit with the realization that as an outspoken, sex-positive reality TV celebrity/nude model/polyamory activist with dozens of artsy naked pictures on the Internet, I was officially no longer parent-friendly material. I had also spent many years identifying with being the polite, graceful, cultured, well-read, and articulate woman that positively charmed the bejesus out of my beau's parents. Now all of those positive qualities had to counterbalance the hefty weight of being a controversial public figure associated with sexuality closely enough that it was uncomfortable at the dinner table.

Maybe you're brand-new and bushy-tailed, excited by the colorful landscape of non-monogamy and all it has to offer. Or maybe you've been happily settled in your chosen polycule for years now, handling jealousy and scheduling conflicts like a champion. Regardless of where you are in the journey, at some point you may have to face a daunting milestone: coming out of the closet.

"But I'm not gay/transgender/queer/bisexual/etc. I don't need to come out of any closet," you might say. Or "I am gay/transgender/queer/bisexual/etc., and I remember when I came out. It sucked!" The proverbial closet belongs not only to these communities, but to anyone who is forced to hide their true nature for fear of negative reactions from family, friends, or the world at large. In the years before the civil rights movement, African Americans who were light-skinned enough to convincingly appear Caucasian could use that to their advantage to land better jobs and avoid much of the harsh stigma leveled at African Americans at that time. This was referred to as "passing," a term that, like "coming out of the closet," has been borrowed by other stigmatized groups.

"Passing" can refer to masculine gay men or feminine lesbians whose appearance and characteristics don't trigger the average person's "gaydar." It may refer to a pre-op transgender individual who passes as their biological sex, or a post-op transgender person who passes as their reassigned gender. The woman who spends her weekends as a dominatrix doling out sweet, sadistic pleasure, but heads to her desk job every Monday morning without a hint of suspicion from her coworkers, could be described as "passing."

Non-monogamous and polyamorous folk may find it relatively easy to "pass" as normal, everyday, monogamous people. If you are opening up a previously established relationship, or if you only introduce one of your partners to your family and friends, it is possible to go for years without anyone knowing a thing. Or you may be able to pass as decidedly single if you don't bring any of your partners home—it's easy to give the impression that you're just dating around and doing your own thing without worrying about settling down.

There are many valid reasons to choose to "pass" as something else rather than coming out of the closet. You may be in a situation where coming out is not worth the risks, or could be physically dangerous to you or those you love. But if there are no immediate threats to your welfare and safety, I urge you to come out and share with the world the joy, love, and fulfillment that you've discovered. In this chapter, you'll come to understand the risks and benefits inherent in being out. You'll also be able to evaluate the best time to come out and how to broach that conversation with the most important people in your life.

Risks

I dream of the day that alternative relationships are no longer considered "alternative." When you can mention to anyone off the street that you are polyamorous, or in an open relationship, or sometimes like to romp around with your swinger friends, and the reaction will be as nonchalant as if you told them about your work as an insurance adjuster. Someday, being in a nontraditional relationship won't dominate the conversation with a lengthy explanation. But until that day, you can expect all kinds of reactions and consequences, some of which will unfortunately be quite negative. At this time, coming out poses a number of risks to be considered.

It can affect your job.

There is an ethical and legal expectation that employers will not discriminate against an employee on the basis of race, religion, gender, age, or sexuality. This expectation stands in the face of a long history full of blatant discrimination against non-whites, non-Westerners, women, transgender and genderqueer people, the elderly, homosexuals, bisexuals, Christians, Muslims, Jews, Buddhists, and yes, even white, cisgender males in some cases.

Sexual or gender-based discrimination in the workplace occupies a particular corner, however. The average cisgender, heterosexual employee may feel comfortable talking about the first date from the night before, going out to lunch with her boyfriend, or the romantic vacation plans she is making for next week, husband, and none of these will give anyone reason to pause. However, someone of an alternative sexuality may never be able to talk about her lifestyle, her partners, or her gender identity, without it being associated with deviancy and abnormality by others. In the past (and sadly in some places around the world today), if one was openly gay, it highlighted the kind of sex one was having and with whom. This person didn't just represent something different, but forced an uncomfortable acknowledgment of sex itself. And though sexual and romantic expression are an inseparable part of human identity, sex and the workplace do not mix.

Similarly, a person who is openly polyamorous at work highlights not the expansive power of love, but rather a way of having sex with multiple people that is far outside the boundaries of "normal." Others may even see it as unethical, flagrant, or completely inappropriate. If you work with children, the reactions will be even more scandalized. The culture of your workplace may be open, accepting, and welcoming, but for many people, being open about polyamory or non-monogamy would be a direct threat to their career.

It may upset your family and friends.

They say that if you ever think you've attained enlightenment, go and spend some time with your family. The people in your family have likely known you since before you were born—probably some of the longest-lasting relationships you've ever had. Long-term relationships inevitably develop their own strengths, weaknesses, neuroses, and lots and lots of history. Your parents and siblings know exactly how to push your buttons for good or ill; not only because they've had years of study, but because they were the ones to install them in the first place.

This is why coming out to your family is an entirely different ballgame. You may be out and proud, not giving a hoot what the rest of the world thinks. But one disapproving comment from your big sister, and you crumple into a ball of doubt and tears. (Yours truly.) You may be able to comfortably discuss relationships and sexuality with your mom, but the thought of broaching that conversation with your dad puts a lump in your throat. For some of us, the approval of our parents is a priceless treasure sought from early childhood, and receiving their disapproval feels like the most crushing of failures.

If your parents, siblings, grandparents, or other close family members disapprove of your choices, it's probably going to hurt, especially if the relationships are healthy and close. But recognize that it's likely to come from a place of love, though it may not feel like it in the moment. These are the people who care for your well-being, who may feel protective of you, and who want you to be happy and successful. If they don't understand your life, your relationships, or what motivates you to make the choices you've made, they may feel that you are making a terrible mistake and only wish to protect you from getting hurt. Poly women in particular often report family members jumping to the conclusion that they are are being taken advantage of and immediately seeking to protect them.

Examine what emotional ties you have to your family's approval or disapproval. These emotional ties may have different levels of intensity for different family members. Being aware of these ties can help you discover whom to prioritize when coming out, and how best to care for yourself if there is a negative reaction.

> When I came out to my mother, she was initially quite upset. "This isn't what I wanted for you," she told me through tears. "I want you to be in a relationship with someone who will love you, who will respect you, who will care for you." I told her about my partners. How wonderful they were, how loved and secure I felt, how I had an abundance of affection and care. I had to reassure her that I actually had all the things that she wanted for me, just in a different shape from what she expected.

You will be passed over for dates and rejected for relationships.

It is undeniable that we're living in a monogamous world. Only 4 percent of the American population openly reports being involved in some form of non-monogamous relationship.[1] Many people choose to stay closeted, so let's be generous and project that as much as 10 percent of the population is currently in or seeking polyamorous or non-monogamous relationships. Assuming that that small portion of the population is happy enough with their experiences so far to continue to pursue non-monogamous relationships, that means one in ten people would be willing to be in a nontraditional relationship with you.

This theoretically implies that if you went on ten first dates with ten different people you met on the street or at the gym or in your dodgeball club, nine of those would not want a second date after you brought up polyamory. So let's say good riddance to those people, and focus on the one person who didn't turn tail at the mention of non-monogamy. Unfortunately, there's still a number of factors that make the odds of finding a good partner worse. This person may want to be a swinger and can't stomach the idea of polyamory. Or you may not be attracted to them whatsoever. Or there could be any number of influences that make the two of you incompatible.

This means that you're likely to field a lot of rejection while seeking out partners. You'll be passed over on dating sites, and you may even receive insulting messages. People who strike up a flirtatious conversation with you at the bar may balk and look mildly nauseated to hear you talk about having other partners. And a new, promising relationship may end in heartbreak once the other person realizes that polyamory is not their cup of tea. To look at this rationally, it really is for the best that people who are not compatible with you move on to someone else who is. But that rationality doesn't take away the sting of being rejected.

But you won't only be on the receiving side of rejection. You will also have to turn down flirtations and relationships. You will encounter people you're attracted to, who are kind and funny and compliment you and make you feel good about yourself, but who you will have to say no to because they want something very different from what you are offering. At the end of the day, your chances of feeling the pain of rejection will increase, and your dating pool will get much smaller.

I don't mention this to be a bummer. If anything, it means that the partners you do find are a rare breed. Even more reason to be ecstatically grateful for them! The fear of rejection, unfortunately, leads people to less-than-savory actions, such as concealing their other partners from a new partner, delivering a sugarcoated description of their lifestyle on a first date, or glossing over the details of their polyamory practice on a dating profile. If you find yourself tempted to do these things, it is better to pull back and reconsider whether your desire for polyamory can outweigh your fear of rejection.

You'll have to explain yourself constantly.

Not only will you be spending time talking with your partners, ironing out agreements and airing your emotions, but you'll be answering the rest of the world's questions about your relationships. And it won't stop there. Conversations about nontraditional relationships will likely give rise to in-depth explanations of your philosophy, your feelings, your religious and political leanings, your worldview, and the nature of love itself. Incidentally, years of doing this have exposed me to every possible question, comment, or argument under the sun about polyamory, and learning to respond effectively has become the foundation for my relationship coaching practice and for the Multiamory podcast.

If you are with people who are genuinely curious, these conversations can be stimulating, informative, and revealing. When you open up about the details of your romantic life, you'll be surprised how many people will open up to you in turn. If you are with people who are scandalized, offended, or otherwise have their hackles up, these conversations may be more of a defensive debate. Ultimately, everybody has an opinion, good or bad, and some people will not be too shy to share it with you before you've asked for it. You will have to learn to field questions and face confrontation with grace.

The custody of your children may be compromised.

This is one of the most painful and frightening issues facing parents who are polyamorous. Sadly, there is already a history of judges revoking child custody because the polyamorous lifestyle of the parents was deemed unsuitable and dangerous. For this reason, most polyamorous people who have children choose to remain in the closet. Because there is still relatively little awareness to distinguish polyamory as a valid lifestyle choice rather than some strange sexual kink, it is all too easy for a judge to believe that children are being exposed to something unhealthy and perverse. Gracie X, author of *Wide Open: My Adventures in Poly-amory, Open Marriage, and Loving On My Own Terms,* was happily living in a duplex with her boyfriend, her husband, her husband's girlfriend, and their four children when Social Services came knocking at their door. Her boyfriend's ex-wife, having learned about their living arrangement, initiated a custody case. Gracie and her family ended up settling out of court, but only after a laborious back and forth, multiple visits and evaluations from social workers, and costly consultations with several lawyers.

Not everyone is as fortunate as Gracie was. Despite the growing body of evidence that being raised in a polyamorous household is not detrimental to children, many courts will easily revoke the custody of parents who are involved in any romantic or sexual behavior perceived to be deviant. If your close family members, or any close adult involved in the lives of your children, are proactively accepting of polyamory, then you may be safe to come out of the closet. If not, losing your children may be too large of a risk.

The Benefits of Coming Out

The risks of coming out may paint a bleak picture, but there is a wealth of ben-efits to be found as well. If the risks outlined above do not apply to you, or are not dire enough to discourage you from being out, then you have many rewards to look forward to, such as the following:

You'll live in honesty and integrity.

The classic truism "Honesty is the best policy" gets tossed around a lot, though few of us are batting a thousand when it comes to practical application. We are frequently dishonest about our true feelings, whether it's avoiding telling our annoying coworker just how irritating she really is or telling your boyfriend how much of a crush you have on his close friend. Even more often, we are dishonest with ourselves about our intentions, our true nature, or what it is we really want out of a relationship. Radical honesty 24/7 is admirable, but also easily offends. Our daily white lies to ourselves and others may both help and hurt us.

Stepping out of the closet offers a refreshing chance to live a more authentic life. At the moment, you may be coming up with all kinds of colorful stories to explain to your parents why you took a weekend trip with someone who isn't your husband. Or you may go so far as to invite multiple romantic partners to a party, but painstakingly avoid any outward displays of affection. If you are not in a safe place to be out, these measures may be necessary, but if you are able to take the vulnerable step of portraying yourself and your life with 100 percent accuracy—no cover-ups, no excuses, no apologies—you will be overwhelmed with a newfound sense of freedom. When you no longer have to worry about keeping lies straight or withholding incriminating information, you are able to live with integrity, feeling like you get to be *you* at any given moment.

It will be easier to find like-minded people.

Clearly spelling out your relationship preferences on a dating profile or to the attractive stranger in the bar will most assuredly receive some rebuffs. But on the flip side, it will be a shining beacon to those who think and feel the same way that you do. The day that I stopped explaining my polyamorous desires in the form of apologies and excuses was a big turning point for me. When I began proudly telling potential dating partners about what I wanted for my relationships, I started finding people who wanted the same exact things.

This isn't just about finding quality partners to date. Being out of the closet also gives you a chance to connect to a community of fellow poly, non-monogamous, or kinky folk who are experiencing the same joys and struggles that you are. It's the first step to having a support network of people who can share your pain, offer a listening ear, or give much-needed advice. Such a support system is priceless, and you can learn more about that in chapter 10.

Your partners can enjoy receiving your attention and love openly.

"I have all of this love and all of this energy and positivity, and I feel like I can't actually put it anywhere," my client Camille lamented to me. She, her husband, her boyfriend, and her boyfriend's wife were not yet out of the closet to their family members or friends for legitimate reasons of safety. Because they were not in a situation where it was safe to be out, Camille could not hold hands with her boyfriend in public, could not be seen with her boyfriend's children, and—the most difficult part for her—could not share how excited and fulfilled she was by her multiple relationships. Others in Camille's situation often have to unintentionally hurt their partners by never mentioning them to family members, avoiding posting pictures together on social media, or telling others that their intensely passionate relationship is just a friendship.

No one likes being hidden. Even if you fully understand your partner's need to be discreet, it is dehumanizing knowing that you virtually do not exist in certain areas of your partner's life. Once you are free from having to hide, omit, protect, or withdraw, your partners get to enjoy you at your fullest, with no reservations. You can reap the benefits of love-affirming actions such as receiving affection in public, being associated on social media, joining social events or family celebrations, and many others.

Who Gets to Know

So you've tallied up all the risks and rewards above and decided that it's time to say good-bye to the closet. Congratulations! Now comes the hard part: figuring out who to tell, when to tell them, and how to tell them.

Gender therapist Dara Hoffman-Fox specializes in helping transgender people come out to family and friends. Years of offering this guidance has led her to create a methodical approach that works well for anything you need to come out of the closet about, including non-monogamy. Hoffman-Fox recommends taking a hard look at the relationships you have with the people you wish to come out to, and her official worksheet actually incorporates tallying up a score for each relationship to determine who in your life needs to be told first. I've adapted her method below, but you can find her full worksheet on her official website, listed in the Resources section.

1. Who do I need to come out to?

Your knee-jerk reaction could be an enthusiastic "Everyone! The whole world!" or a shuddering "Ugh, nobody, please. No one needs to know my secret shame." But let's try to focus between those two extremes. Your list will likely include the people that you interact with on a personal level on a daily basis—certain family members, your best friend, maybe coworkers. In this preliminary stage, some people may be ambiguous. Do you need to come out to your old friends from your hometown you only see a few times a year? If you're unsure, put them on the list anyway.

2. What type of relationship do I have with this person?

For each name you write down, examine the quality of relationship you have. Hoffman-Fox recommends assigning a numerical value to the closeness of the relationship, but it may be more accessible to you to write out brief descriptions. Are you very close with your mom, able to share anything except matters pertaining to sex? Maybe you don't know your new coworker very intimately, but the two of you have connected over open-minded conversations on philosophy, past relationships, or human rights. Cover the main points of these relationships succinctly; don't worry about writing a whole novel (though taking a full, thorough inventory of your personal relationships is a revealing exercise all on its own!).

3. How much do I value this relationship in my life?

Think about what each relationship adds to or subtracts from your life. Your dad may get under your skin at times, but his unfailing support and excellent advice has gotten you out of several scrapes in the past. Alternately, you may enjoy hanging out with your best friend, but her heavy-handed criticism of your personal life may leave you with a bad taste in your mouth after you part ways. Think about how much your life would be affected if any one of these relationships were to dissolve. The absence of certain relationships may not even cause you to bat an eye, while the loss of others would be totally devastating.

4. What am I willing to do to preserve this relationship?

The coming-out conversation can generate a whole range of unexpected reactions. In an ideal world, everyone you know and love would embrace and celebrate your coming out. But few of us are lucky enough to experience such a thing, so it is important to account for the effort that may be necessary to maintain a relationship with someone who reacts negatively to your romantic life. For those relationships in your list that are highly valued, what are the specific actions you are willing to take in order to preserve the relationship? This might mean taking the time to gather and forward educational resources, having the patience to have many, many conversations and answer many, many questions, and the willingness to listen to this person who may express negative feelings to you. On the other hand, this can also reveal which relationships have lower stakes, which may subsequently relieve you from worrying about the outcome of a possible negative reaction.

Timing is Everything

Once you've determined who is at the top of your list, it's time to pick a date for having the conversation. This might be motivated by practicalities. If you know you want to bring two of your partners to Thanksgiving, it's necessary that everyone who will be coming to dinner be aware of what's going on. You might want to give it at least a week or two beforehand to have that conversation with the appropriate people. Waiting until you ring the doorbell with your paramours in tow is daring, but likely to be disruptive and potentially damaging.

If you don't have an external event dictating when you need to come out, you are free to set a date on your own. Pick a time frame that has you coming out sooner rather than later. When choosing your time frame, be considerate of the context the other person will be in. It's best to avoid hijacking a day that may be very important to this person in order to talk about yourself (e.g. their wedding). It's best if you can find a time to sit down with this person one-on-one in a place where you're both comfortable and are unlikely to be interrupted. Some people choose a personal space such as the person's own home for the level of privacy and comfort it provides, though others prefer finding a public space such as a low-key coffee shop in order to curtail over-the-top emotional reactions. You will have to make this choice depending on the person you are coming out to.

Born This Way?

For years, there was ongoing debate over the nature of homosexuality. Religious groups asserted that it was a choice, albeit a misguided one sure to lead to fiery punishment in the afterlife. Psychologists long held that it was a mental disorder—a case of developmental crossed wires, leading one astray from normal, healthy sexual attraction to the opposite sex. Other conservative sets still insist that it's a conspiracy, the destructive desires of sexual deviants seeking to corrupt others and continually push the "gay agenda." But within the past few decades, there has been increasing evidence that homosexuality is the result of genetic and environmental factors, far outside the realm of a conscious decision. It is unlikely that you would be able to pinpoint a precise moment when you decided what your sexuality would be; it is more likely that you just knew from a very early age who was attractive to you and who wasn't. The general mentality around homosexuality is in the process of shifting—from a story of mental illness and deviancy to one of acceptance and understanding.

As of this writing, there has not been an adequate amount of research to determine if there is such a thing as a "polyamory gene." Who knows what scientists would even look for? A common genetic marker in people who desire many sex partners? A particular sequence that switches on the capacity to fall in love with more than one person at the same time? A gene dedicated to managing scheduling conflicts? Some argue that the natural state of human beings is to be non-monogamous, so would it be more appropriate to look for a monogamy gene? Should they try to find the trait that leaves some people predisposed to uncompromising jealousy and others total junkies for compersion?

Science has yet to offer definitive answers, so we are left to conjecture and anecdotes. I've heard some people describe discovering polyamory like a homecoming—finding the validation and acceptance for thoughts and feelings that began in very early childhood. Other people feel more like a "switch"—no strong leanings to be either monogamous or non-monogamous, but content with whatever format their relationship is taking at that exact moment. For some, this is their identity, and for others, just a practical approach to relationships that happens to work best for them right now.

This can affect the way people react to you when you tell them about your relationships. If you've inwardly felt a desire for multiple partners your entire life, you may be hurt when people condemn you for choosing something they consider to be aberrant and unnatural. Alternately, you may be put off if this is something that works for you right now but someone treats you like you've got an inescapable predisposition to sex addiction or an inherent inability to commit to a relationship.

The Conversation

There is no single formula for the perfect coming-out conversation. Each relationship you have is different, with unique history and dynamics. The approach you take with your best friend will be different from the approach you take with your grandparents. To have the most effective coming-out conversations, regardless of who it is with, remember these three things:

1. Be educated and experienced.

Make sure that you've done your homework. Read polyamory blogs, forum posts, and books like this one. Know your facts about sexual health. You probably already did this kind of research when first considering a non-monogamous relationship, but it helps to expose yourself to a variety of opinions and interpretations to fill in the gaps. It may be useful to review the common misconceptions covered in chapter 1. No book will contain answers for every possible question you might get asked, but having more information rather than less will instill you with confidence heading in.

It's also important to have a little bit of experience under your belt. Wait at least a month after beginning to pursue a polyamorous lifestyle before coming out to those who are most likely to be skeptical. A former partner of mine came out to her mother and her closest friends immediately after deciding to open up her relationship, but before she and her boyfriend had actually tried dating anyone else. She received several negative reactions, and she was unable to uphold that it was working for her relationship and making her happy, because she genuinely had no idea if it even would yet! Being able to speak from actual experience demonstrates your commitment to trying out this change, and it lends you credibility as well.

2. Be calm.

Yes, you might be heading into one of the most intimidating conversations of your life, and I'm telling you to be calm. Depending on who you are coming out to, there will naturally be some level of nervousness, but do your best to care for yourself in such a way that you can maintain a level head during the conversation. When I was coming out to my aunt and uncle, whose opinion I cared very much about, I was so nervous that I downed two strong cocktails faster than I had ever consumed any drink in my life. I got decidedly tipsy in about five minutes and struggled to talk about my relationships in an articulate and intelligent-sounding way. There are many ways to avoid my mistake: try meditating, getting in some exercise, or even having an orgasm earlier in the day. All of these are proven to reduce the jitters and help you think more clearly when heading into a tense situation.

If the person you're talking to has a negative or emotionally intense reaction, it is imperative that you maintain your inner calm. Give this person their space to react and to process, but do not escalate the situation by matching their emotional level. Avoid raising your voice, making physical displays of agitation, or letting the conversation stray from the realm of discussion and into the gladiatorial arena. Regardless of what you say, the other person may remain upset and disapproving. As hard as it may be to walk away from the conversation when someone you care about is upset with you, it will be much better for that relationship in the long run if you keep your cool, instead of fighting tooth and nail to change this person's mind.

3. Be happy.

People may argue the fine points and logistics of your lifestyle. They may tell you that you are sinful, dirty, crazy, confused, sick, or just plain wrong. They may insult you or your partners. But at the end of the day, no one can argue with your happiness. No one can tell you what you are feeling inside. If the person you are coming out to incessantly argues with you about your life and refuses to drop it, it may be time to calmly state, "I understand and appreciate your concerns. Rest assured that the choices I've made are currently making me very happy." Then walk away from the conversation and keep on pursuing that happiness. (If you cannot truthfully say to the other person that you are happy with your relationships, it is probably not the time to be coming out of the closet.)

Coming Out to a Partner

Some people come to the realization that they are polyamorous while in the middle of a monogamous relationship. It's exciting to find a relationship philosophy that resonates with you, but terrifying to face the prospect of having that conversation with your monogamous partner. Here are a few tips to keep in mind:

- **Find a nonthreatening entry point.** Rather than hopping straight to "I want to open our relationship," lead with a soft opener. It might be "I stumbled onto this podcast about polyamory. Really fascinating stuff. How do you feel about that?" Or you could try being a little more direct. "Can we talk about what it might be like to be in an open relationship?"
- **Know what you want.** Before the conversation, have a clear idea of what is appealing to you about non-monogamy. Is it the sexual variety? Is it the idea of having multiple coparents someday? Is it the opportunity to play with your partner in a group sex situation?
- **Emphasize inclusion.** Make sure your partner knows that this is not something you want to do against his will or without his consent. Emphasize that this is a journey you will take together, and that you are supportive of his individual dating life as well.

- **Be mindful of terminology.** You may not be totally aware of the connotations or associations your partner has with particular vocabulary. If you toss out the terms "polyamory" or "open relationship," follow up with explanations of exactly what that means to you.
- **Discuss everything, but accept that you can't plan for all contingencies.** Discuss your boundaries and agreements, but understand that unexpected situations can and will arise. Make a commitment to flexibility, and establish trust that you will be able to talk things out regardless of what happens.
- **Offer to let your partner go first.** If it feels right to you, let your partner take the first step, such as being the first to create a dating profile or the first to go out on a date. Demonstrate your support of your partner's dating life, and be the most compassionate version of yourself you can be.

Reactions to Coming Out

❝My mother and I are very close but it was almost a year before I could tell her, because I was scared of her reaction. Initially it was rough, she cried, said I was ruining my marriage, asked why I bothered to get married in the first place, and hung up on me. Thankfully that was not the end of the conversation; she kept talking to me about it and slowly has become more accepting. Last summer she came up to visit and met my husband's girlfriend; by the end she was calling her 'my other daughter.' She listens and asks questions when she needs to, she seems happy for me, and has stated that she sees that I am happier than I have ever been, and that this style of relationship seems to work for me.❞ —Bria

❝I'm not 'out' about being poly, or having any relationships and orientations other than 'straight woman married to straight dude,' in my offline public life. My parents don't know and have both made actively hateful remarks about polyamory and LGBT any time it has come up on a television special . . . so they aren't going to know, ever, if I have anything to say about it. My partners are totally in agreement with me about this, and none of them wishes to meet my relatives.❞ —Mia

❝I was spending a few months the year after I graduated college working for my dad at his architecture/construction company managing the front desk and the office. A friend of mine from college was working on his application to medical school and needed someone to proofread it for him. Part of his essay included that he's Chinese and lives in a very traditional home but he's gay and his family didn't know. What I didn't know was that

I had saved the file to the desktop on my work computer and my dad found it. Skimming the first paragraph and not much else, apparently, he came to the conclusion that I was gay and didn't know how to tell him. He went and talked to his psychologist, he spent nights awake thinking about it, processing it, and coming to the conclusion that he loves me and accepts me the way that I am. He calls me, sounding grave, and asks to take me to dinner to talk about something. I accept and tell him that I have stuff to talk about with him as well. He starts and tells me, 'Sweetie, I found your essay on the work computer. I know, and I want you to know that I love you.' And I say, 'What essay? Hubert's med school application?' He was confused for a good minute while the waitress came up and brought us drinks. When she finally leaves, he says, 'Wait, so you're not gay?' I just laughed and told him that I'm also not Chinese. Even though I'm not gay, he wanted me to know that he would accept me and love me the same even if I was. Telling him about polyamory after that was easy. He told me the same principle still applies and that as long as it makes me happy, he doesn't care what I do. He still supports me and even tells other people about it and answers their questions and stuff. It's adorable. **"** —Brooke

Chapter 9 Homework

Exercise #1

If you haven't already, make your priority list of who to come out to. (A+ students will fill out Dara Hoffman-Fox's whole worksheet.) Before jumping in, take your list to someone you trust and who you are already out to. An outsider's perspective can cast new light on the best people to approach and how to approach them. Siblings, in particular, offer excellent insight for approaching parents, for example.

Exercise #2

You won't always get the luxury of having an hours-long conversation with everyone you come out to. If you're in a context that doesn't allow for elaborate explanation, it helps to come up with a condensed version of your coming-out speech. Most people prioritize communicating that their relationships involve mutual consent, honesty, and transparency. Your priorities may be different. If you had to give a thirty-second "elevator pitch" version of your relationship dynamics, what would it be?

❤10 Finding Your Tribe

When I made my first online dating profile, I was brand-new to poly-amory but quite eager to dive in and see what it was all about. My boyfriend at the time had only reluctantly agreed and was reticent to even discuss any details or negotiate any agreements, which in hindsight should have been a red flag. But I was chomping at the bit, feeling like a kid who just got handed a new toy. Within a matter of days after officially opening our relationship, I was all signed up on a popular dating website, delighted by the flood of attention I was already receiving in my inbox.

Despite the high interest, it was difficult fielding rejection and skepticism about my open relationship. This was in 2011, and the online presence of poly-amory was still gaining ground. Initially, I was excited when I started receiving rare messages from others who also identified as non-monogamous. *I've found my people!* I would think. Though that excitement fell when I realized that "my people" were, frankly, quite weird.

There was the man whose profile was all pictures of him and his girlfriend dressed in *Tron* cosplay, the professional Dom who insisted that our first date be at a BDSM club, the purple-haired woman who was interested in dating me, but only if I could have sex with her boyfriend too (she made sure to send dick pics for my convenience). I so desperately wanted to belong, wanted to eat at the cool-poly-kids table, but I was completely put off. *Who the heck are all these weirdos? Is this what the polyamory community looks like? What have I gotten myself into?*

After several years of running in this circle, I've come to learn that the alternative attracts people from all walks of life. Going against the grain is not for the faint of heart, and those who have already made the leap out of the mainstream are usually quite comfortable embracing other things that are off the beaten path—BDSM, gender-fuckery, political anarchy, experimental art, and every flavor of sci-fi enthusiast, anime fan, hardcore gamer, and fantasy nerd. (None of this, by the way, is expressed in the pejorative. My own nerd roots run quite deep.)

So when you envision the polyamorous community at large, know that it embraces a wide range of folk, from the everyman to the extremist, from vanilla to hot sauce. And also know that once you dive into the world of non-monogamy, it is this community that you'll be stepping into, like it or not.

Community vs. Tribe

Honestly, the word "community" makes me twitch. It conjures up visions of people smiling through gritted teeth as they accept a serving of their neighbor's infamously flavorless potluck dish. The community bulletin board where you can find passive-aggressive requests to "please pick up your dog's poop, you know who you are." The neighborhood clean-up day that no one looks forward to.

I'm more enamored with the word "tribe." Human beings started out in tribes. It was the first social structure we ever knew! In early human history, you were likely to have grown up in a group of anywhere from thirty to 150 people. Many of these people would have known you since you were born and would have helped feed you and care for you when you were sick. In turn, you would be present for the birth and growth of every new member of the tribe, witnessing their good moments and bad. Unless you encountered another tribe, you would spend most of your days without running into anyone you could call a stranger. You ate, slept, hunted, and mated with people that you already knew. More details on this can be found in chapter 2.

After millennia of cultural shift, blending, and upheaval, the Agrarian and Industrial revolutions, and the effects of wars, politics, and technological developments, our daily social lives have taken on an entirely different shape. The nuclear family unit is paramount, semi-penetrable from the outside only by those who legally marry into it. (Even then, trying to blend with a family of in-laws is no walk in the park.) We are more likely to spend our days surrounded by strangers, or at best acquaintances, punctuated by interactions with just a few people intimately close to us. It is a confusing experience, disquieting to our deeply buried human instincts—to be surrounded by other humans, yet still capable of feeling alienated and profoundly alone.

Short of a global catastrophe, it is unlikely we'll return to our simpler days of kicking it around the campfire with the rest of the tribe. But even the most reclusive and introverted shut-in still relies on the presence of other people in order to survive. We eagerly or begrudgingly sign up for online social networks. Ultimately, most of us are more likely to seek intimate relationships and friendships rather than become solitary hermits. We are still trying to get back to that campfire.

Whatever word you choose, the people who make up your inner circle, your community, your tribe are the people who sustain you, support you, love you, and bring you more fully into the experience of being human. It is possible to keep your relationships compartmentalized—making sure certain partners don't meet your family, your friends, or each other—but I've yet to meet anyone who wasn't totally miserable doing this. The more cohesion and peace present in your tribe, the more happiness for everyone in it.

Chosen Family

Most of us may not have been born into a full-blown tribe, but all of us entered the world with some kind of family ties. You may love the family that you were born into, or you may loathe them with every fiber of your being. Unfortunately, no one came to you beforehand and asked, "How do you feel about having a sassy but compassionate grandmother?" or "Would you like to have an alcoholic father or no?" For better or worse, you have to take the cards you were dealt.

But the concept of family extends beyond genetic ties. Your tribe, your pod, your group, your support network, your polycule is your *chosen* family. These are the people who have entered your life that you have chosen to make part of your inner circle. You have actively chosen to bring these people near to you, to accept the ups and downs, experience the ecstatic joys and bothersome frustrations that are inherent to human connections.

Your chosen family may include the friends you've had since elementary school, your roommate, your partners, your metamours, and a collection of mutual friends that you share. If you are in a triad or a quad, where all partners are involved with one another, the foundation of your chosen family may be just that. Or you may be happiest in a close network of multiple dyads, where you feel comfortable chilling with your metamours and calling the whole gang together for the occasional board game night.

Looking for Love

I've had numerous clients reach out to me, exclaiming, "I've decided to try poly-amory! I'm so excited! But I live in a small town . . . how the heck do I find people to date?" or "I keep getting turned down. I can't take this rejection! Where do all the poly people hang out?" It naturally follows that once you've decided to change your approach to dating and relationships, you're probably raring to go out and actually take it for a spin. If you picked up this book, it's unlikely your number one concern was how to find more poly-friendly *acquaintances* (though I'll discuss that later in the chapter).

Modern-day courtship is a beast of its own, for better or worse. While sexual minorities once had to rely on specialized physical locations (think Dyke Night down at the dive bar, or gay bathhouse culture), the Internet has revolutionized how we find dating partners that are compatible with our preferences and ideologies. Some people make a fuss about this, mourning the loss of the days when you might meet an attractive and mysterious stranger in a bar and flirt until the sun comes up, getting to know each other the "natural" way. I am all in favor of going after organic opportunities and letting yourself be open to an unplanned and unexpected rendezvous, but it's also a drag when the attractive and mysterious stranger you've been flirting with all night lets it drop that she would never consider a non-monogamous relationship of any kind, that her political beliefs are diametrically opposed to yours, and she thinks that homosexuality is a birth defect caused by all the chemicals in fast food. (True story.)

Some people love dating. They love the stimulation of meeting someone new, delighting in the dance of flirtation and conversation. Others find dating to be a total drag. They dread the whole rigmarole of getting dressed up and exchanging polite conversation, feeling nervous if they like the other person, and feeling awkward if they don't. Whatever your stance, polyamory is still on the fringe, which kicks up the difficulty level on dating and partner-seeking. Most people you would meet out on the street are expecting that any serious connection will naturally lead to monogamy, and the parameters and requirements for a non-monogamous relationship are an instant deal breaker. You can find specific statistics on this in chapter 9. Many people get around this by turning to online dating to find like-minded partners. Online dating is far from perfect, but it expedites the process of filtering good or bad matches by allowing for total transparency up front. It can also be helpful to connect to a local polyamory meet-up group to find dating partners who are already experienced in non-monogamy. (More on meet-up groups later in this chapter.)

Regardless of where and how you seek partners, there are three important things to bring to your dating practice: transparency, authenticity, and flexibility.

Transparency

First and foremost, you need to be up-front about the fact that you are not seeking monogamy, and are unlikely to seek it with anyone in the future. Be specific about how you identify or what kind of relationship style you subscribe to (Polyamory? Swinging? Relationship anarchist? Consensual non-monogamy?). And because you're at the mercy of any number of preconceived notions about polyamory or non-monogamy, give details about what your relationship choice *means* to you. Talk about what you're looking for, how many other partners you have, and how important those relationships are to you.

If you're making an online dating profile, it's up to you whether these details go at the beginning, middle, or end. I usually give a brief description at the very beginning of my profile, then go more in depth later on. I've even included a Van Halen–inspired catch: buried in the middle of my profile, I request that any message sent to me include the phrase "Green M&Ms." If I get a message without green M&Ms in it, I know the person didn't fully read my profile.

If you're pursuing dating partners offline, the basics of this information should be conveyed before the first date even happens. No need to launch into your full spiel the moment that you meet, but the earlier that this person knows you are non-monogamous, the better.

This may seem like a lot of information to give right out of the gate. However, the more detailed information you are able to give a potential dating partner, the better she will be able to give or withhold her consent to entering a dating relationship with you. The key here is that she will be able to give *informed* consent—she knows what to expect from you, what the shape of your life is, and with an understanding of all the factors in play, she can give a solid "yes" or "no."

The terrifying specter of "no" is what drives us to sugarcoat information. To gloss over certain uncomfortable details, to make only vague allusions to our other relationships, or even to choose to omit information about the existence of our other partners entirely. This tactic works great in the short term. But in the long term, the truth about your life becomes harder and harder to cover up, and it becomes more and more likely that both you and this other person will get hurt. Transparency up front may be uncomfortable, but it saves you from a world of pain down the line.

Authenticity

The more transparency you have, the more authentic you become. Authenticity comes from your outward presentation coming into congruent alignment with your inner self. When you meet someone new and exciting and you're feeling that hint of a spark, you can feel the peace that comes from knowing that they *see* you, wholly, stripped of artifice and pretense. When you are operating authentically, you can dive into the great joy of being loved holistically.

Be warned: this is a lifelong pursuit. As nice as authenticity sounds, it is freaking *hard*. When you're heading into a first date, you want that person to like you, to accept you. If you like that person enough to go on date number two and number three, you *really* want that person to like you, and the stakes start creeping higher. No one wants to expose themselves, crying, "This is me and this is the shape of my life. This is 100 percent bona fide authentic me!" and have the other person take a look, purse their lips, and say, "Um, thanks, but no thanks." The very idea of it makes us want to collapse into a withered pile of hurt feelings and bruised ego.

In her book *If the Buddha Dated,* Charlotte Kasi describes the way we put on masks at the beginning of relationships. We put on the masks of charm, of attractiveness, of wit, of any number of elaborate facades in order to make us look more appealing. The tragedy comes when, later on, you are faced with the choice to either to wear the mask for the rest of your life, or to remove the mask and risk losing someone you love because you no longer match their expectations of you.

The eternal challenge is to acknowledge the fear of being authentic and choose to be authentic anyway. It can take a long time to break the habit of trotting out your collection of masks on every date, but with a firm commitment to authenticity, the number of masks in your collection gets pared down over time.

Flexibility

Even if you're batting a thousand on transparency and authenticity, things may still not work out in the end. That funny, attractive, irresistibly charming person who was on board with polyamory from the get-go may go on a first date with you and come to the conclusion that it's just not for him. Or he may come to this conclusion after you've been dating for six months, after you've developed feelings for each other. You may send online messages to any number of non-monogamy-friendly folk who seem like they would be just *perfect* for you, and never receive a response.

The process of finding partners is always going to have some disappointments, and the only way to make it through without banging your head against the wall is to have flexibility. If you create a rigidly defined box that potential partners have to perfectly fit into, it's likely you will be disappointed by all the people that don't fit. Some people launch into the world of dating with a laundry list—"She has to be bisexual and equally attracted to both me and my partner," or "He has to never disagree with any of my opinions and never get upset with anything I do," or "He has to be at least three inches taller than me."

The reality is that people are not box-shaped. They change and grow and shift constantly. The person who seems to tick all the boxes on your list may not be suited for you five years down the line, and the person you meet today who is lacking some of your requirements may turn out to fulfill you in ways you didn't even imagine were possible. Non-monogamy allows you to relax the box mentality. You aren't looking for the one perfect person who will fit you today, tomorrow, and fifty years from now, which means you get the great opportunity to expand the limits of what you look for in a romantic partner.

Of course, if the person you're on a date with declares that she will be monogamous into eternity, there are going to be some fundamental problems. But outside of direct and obvious incompatibilities, let yourself be present and let yourself be flexible. Head into your date without expectations, positive or negative, and allow yourself to enjoy connecting with another being, sharing a conversation and a brief moment in time, and then continuing on your own way, open to however the future between you may unfold.

Know When to Say Yes, Know When to Say No, Know When to Ask the Question

The "No Means No" campaign generated awareness around consent and sexual assault. The slogan highlighted that if a woman says "no" to a sexual encounter, it doesn't mean she's playing hard to get, it doesn't mean she's too proud to say yes, it doesn't mean that she is afraid of coming across as easy. It just means no.

Many institutions later swapped this for "Yes means yes!", shifting the focus to encourage people to express positive, ongoing consent during sexual encounters. In both sex and relationships, it is important to know when to say no and when to say yes. But as important as these campaigns are, they also perpetuate the assumption that women are always the ones responding to the question, never the ones asking it.

The traditional dating game thrives on equally traditional gender roles. Women are brought up to be passive participants in the arenas of dating and sex, responding to the advances made by men who are brought up to be the proactive initiators. Anyone who has spent time on a mainly heterosexual online dating site can witness this dynamic at play. Men spend their time crafting messages ranging from the simple to the elaborate, the low-key to the borderline desperate. Some men send messages en masse, casting a wide net to balance out the low likelihood that anyone will respond. In the meantime, women are slogging through an ever-filling inbox of messages, many of them well-meaning, some of them downright crude, most of them unwanted.

Offline dating doesn't fare much better. Women primp and doll up, hoping that they'll catch the eye of the attractive gentleman across the room, and posture themselves in such a way that he'll be enticed to come over and make the first move. A man's "game" is supposed to be direct and aggressive. It's expected that the man will be the one to start the conversation, to be the one to ask the woman out on a date, possibly to be the person who takes charge in initiating sex. A woman's "game" is supposed to be coy and subtle. Lots of hints and indirect signals. As one woman once told me, "I would never ask a man out, even if I liked him. If he knows that you like him from the beginning, he holds all the power. You can't let that happen. Have to keep him guessing." To my astonishment, the other women in the conversation wholeheartedly agreed with her.

Further, women are encouraged to be the detached gatekeepers of sex. There's a lot of stock and worry put into when a woman should let a man have sex with her. Is it after the third date? After three months? Whatever happens, the general consensus is that it should *definitely* not be on the first date, not if you don't want him to think that you're a loose and lusty strumpet, far from relationship material.

Where did we learn this? It may be the result of a culture still clinging to the remnants of the days when a woman's virginity and reputation were her most valuable commodities. There is still the threat of slut-shaming, which discourages women from showing too much of an interest in sex, let alone taking steps to actively pursue it. Or maybe, after centuries of disempowerment, we grow up learning very quickly that these head games and carrot-dangling behaviors restore some illusion of power and control.

It is time for us to grow up and cut the crap.

Playing games, dropping hints, and tiptoeing around what you actually want may put you in a less vulnerable position, but it also increases the chances that the object of your affections will be confused, frustrated, or oblivious to what you want. If you are attracted to someone and want to go out on a date with him, tell him you like his style and ask him out for a glass of wine. If you've been flirting with a girl for ages and want nothing more than to roll around in bed with her, get her enthusiastic consent, and then go nuts. If you like someone, as in, *like*-like him, then let him know. Yes, this will open you up to the possibility of vulnerability and rejection, but it also opens you up to the even better possibility of getting what you want, whether that's a hot date, exciting sex, or a deep emotional exchange with the person you've been crushing on for ages.

Cowboys

Finding new partners is an exhilarating and nerve-racking process. The first few dates are flavored with the anticipating of trying someone on, feeling out the chemistry, seeing if expectations align. Sometimes you hit it off from the first moment, discovering that you want and expect the same things from each other, and you get to enjoy the giddy process of drawing close to another human being. Sometimes the vibe is just not there. The conversation doesn't flow, the attraction is missing, or you want entirely different things out of each other. Time to say "thank you for the lovely evening" and move on to greener pastures. But sometimes expectations are ambivalent, especially if you are someone's first exposure to non-monogamy. Enter the "cowboy." (Or cowgirl. Or cow-person.)

The cowboy is someone who has never been in a polyamorous relationship before. He may listen politely as you describe your other partners, your enjoyment of non-monogamy, your alternative philosophy about love, sex, and relationships. He may ask a lot of questions and seem genuinely curious about the way you run your life. After the first date, he'll be intrigued enough to go for date number two, and as time progresses, you may feel a sense of relief that even though he's never tried non-monogamy before, he's found you charming enough to dive in and figure it out for himself.

In reality, the cowboy has an agenda, though he himself may not be consciously aware of it. He'll assume that you're just taking your time to play the field, to explore your options, to enjoy being single for a while before settling down. He'll feel confident that once your relationship with him gets to the right level of emotional intimacy, you'll be ready to forgo all other lovers and enter a monogamous relationship with him. The worst part is that cowboys are rarely up-front about these assumptions. Instead, the truth doesn't come to light until much later, after there's emotional investment on both sides. Eventually, the cowboy realizes that you aren't willing to give up your other relationships and become exclusive with him, and what inevitably follows is frustration, upset, and heartbreak.

Cowboys and cowgirls are not bad people. It is unlikely that the cowgirl sits alone in a dark room, twiddling her fingers like a Bond villain and cackling about her master plan to entrap you. It's doubtful that she sees you as a person unworthy of respect, or that your needs and wants are invalid. Instead, cowboys and cowgirls are the product of a culture that doesn't see non-monogamy as a viable choice for a long-term relationship. Having multiple partners may be okay in the in-between, but when it's time to settle down, you better straighten up and fly right, buddy. This is where things get lost in translation. You say "I'm polyamorous" and the cowgirl hears "I'm dating around." You say "I have multiple romantic partners" and the cowgirl hears "I'll be ready for an exclusive relationship later down the road."

How to avoid cowboys and cowgirls? Most of it is transparency. If you avoid obscuring the details of your relationships and what you're seeking, it automatically filters out most people who would be seeking the exact opposite. It's helpful to go one step further and establish that this is different from being single and playing the field. You may still encounter a cowgirl who, despite your clear communication, will be steadfast in her belief that she can change you. But if you've given 100 percent of your effort to being honest and transparent, she will have to either change her expectations, or avoid a relationship with you. It hurts to see people go, but you'll both be much, much happier.

Of course, cowboy-ing is not exclusive to monogamous folk. Some polyamorists drag out relationships with the die-hard monogamous under the same delusional thinking. I know this because I tried to pull this stunt in several relationships in my early days of poly. I could see so many red flags that it wasn't going to work out, that we wanted different things, and could even be told point-blank by my new partner that he wanted to be monogamous. Still, I would think, "He's just unenlightened. Once he sees what an awesome partner I am, and how great polyamory is, he'll be hooked and everything will go swimmingly!" At the same time, my partner would counter-cowboy me, hopeful that I would abandon my licentious ways and see the light. Sadly, the trope from spaghetti westerns rings true: nobody wins in a standoff.

Poly-prenticing

Some people make a commitment to only date people who already identify as polyamorous, or who are already in a solid non-monogamous relationship or two. This does save a lot of potential frustration and heartbreak, and it's a surefire way to stave off potential cowboys. However, the non-monogamous dating pool is already small, even in large, liberal cities. For those who live in smaller communities or more conservative cultures, this kind of commitment may not be realistic. If you are having a hard time finding fellow polyamorists to date, consider opening yourself up to those outside of the non-monogamous community.

This absolutely requires those three gems: transparency, authenticity, and flexibility. It also requires a wary eye for anyone trying to cowboy you and the ability to take a reality check and make sure that you're not trying to cowboy someone in turn.

So you've weeded out the unwavering monogamous, and you've found yourself flirting with an alluring, open-minded individual who is genuinely curious to know you better and learn what this polyamory thing is all about. It's time to take on an apprentice. Or a poly-prentice.

It will be your responsibility to introduce this person to the world of non-monogamy, which is no mean feat. At the beginning, it will feel like a student-teacher dynamic. Your new partner will be asking most of the questions, and you'll be the one providing most of the answers. In time, it's important to encourage your new partner to explore on their own, do their own research, dive into some reading, go on dates of their own, and practice open communication about their desires, expectations, and other relationships.

There's some debate about whether it's better to ease in someone who is new to polyamory or whether you should toss them into the deep end of the pool. It is your call to make, depending on the individual. I'm in favor of encouraging your new paramour to play with the big kids rather than wading in the kiddie pool. One of my partners makes a specific effort early on in a poly-prenticing relationship to invite any new partner to a house party, where this new partner is likely to meet his friends, coworkers, and his other partners. Some people think this is an excellent, low-pressure way of introducing some-one new into their little tribe; others think the sparrow method (booting them straight out of the nest so they'll learn to fly on the way down) is too intense. Again, it's up to you to decide the most appropriate method to take.

How Many Partners Should You Have?

A classic interview question for poly folk: how many partners are you allowed to have?

As though there were a Polyamory Board of Directors who reviews individual cases and delineates the maximum number of partners each person is allowed.

The number of partners you have depends on the shape of your life, your time constraints, and what it is you're seeking. It's easier to have a greater number of partners if you are seeking relationships that don't require a lot of time commitment, but it becomes harder to have multiple partners if you are focused on building deep connections and spending lots of time with each person. Again, it all depends on what resources and reserves you have to give.

However many partners you choose to have, it's important to main-tain a sense of when you might be *polysaturated*—the point where it may be difficult to add more relationships without compromising the time, energy, and effort given to others.

Cross-poly-nation

If you stick around in a particular location for long enough, you'll find that the poly community can feel incestuous. There are unspoken rules about not dating friends, or friend's exes, or exes' friends, or whatever combination. But in many poly circles, the relatively small dating pool leads some to toss these rules out the window. This is both good and bad. Good, because usually the most popular people in any given poly scene are likely to be quality—demonstrably honest, genuine, supportive of non-monogamy, and good partners. Why else would everyone be drawn to them? Bad, because this is fertile ground for gossip, internal drama, and many toes vulnerable to being stepped on.

Cross-pollination within your inner circle of partners and friends is neither to be categorically avoided nor forced. Whether or not it feels right to date within your inner circle has to be taken on a case-by-case basis. If you find yourself hopelessly attracted to your partner's ex or close friend or even one of his other partners, make the time to check in with everyone's thoughts and feelings before proceeding. Your guiding light should be avoiding any appearance of going behind your partner's back or having no consideration for anyone else's feelings. Lay out a good foundation by talking everything out proactively and inclusively before making any sudden moves.

Connecting to the Community

The landscape of the non-monogamous community at large is expanding day by day. The Internet has made it easier not only to find dating partners, but to find a whole world of other like-minded people. I encourage any client of mine who is brand-new to polyamory to find a meet-up group in their area as soon as possible, but not for the purpose of finding someone to date right away. Many polyamory mixers involve discussion groups or book clubs, where you'll have a chance to ask any questions you may have and share your concerns, or even your excitement and successes. Most importantly, being around other normal poly folk gives you a chance to see just that: normal poly folk, of all ages, shapes, classes, races, and creeds. There will usually be a healthy mix of old hats and total newbies. If your only experience of non-monogamy has been from reading books or browsing online forums, connecting to others face-to-face humanizes the experience. You can find poly meet-up groups in nearly every major city with some quick searching on the Internet and social media.

Your support network may also include poly- and kink-friendly professionals such as therapists, counselors, coaches, and others. Some traditional therapists and mental health professionals pathologize non-monogamous lifestyles, so it's important to seek help that will be understanding and accepting of your relationship choices. You can find links to extensive online directories of open-minded professionals in the Resources section.

Meeting Your Metamours

Your partner's other partners are part of your partner's chosen family, and it is crucial to be on good terms with them. Being on good terms does not mean that you need to have sexual or romantic relationships with your metamours. It does not mean that you need to be best friends, or that you need to feel 100 percent comfortable around them 100 percent of the time. If anyone is pressuring you to have the kind of relationship or interaction with your metamour that you don't want to have, it's time to say something.

Being on good terms means that there should be some sort of connection between you and your metamour. I encourage you to make an effort to reach out to your metamour. If you don't know her already, be the one to make first contact. It doesn't have to be an elaborate introduction, nor does it require pomp and circumstance. This could be as simple as sending a text message to say, "Hi there! Nice to meet you. Let's grab coffee/tea/a beer sometime!" Simple, warm, and effective.

When is the right time to reach out to your partner's new partner? Before the first date is too soon; six months in is too late. I usually wait until I've gotten a sense that this new person is likely to stick around in my partner's life for the time being. If I'm unsure, I ask my partner what his feelings are about the new relationship. If you are the new partner in question, the same guideline applies. Once you've realized that you like this person enough to dive in and see where it goes, it's a good time to meet his chosen family (which includes his other partners).

I'd recommending meeting face-to-face with your metamour at least once. This may not be feasible if your partner is in a long-distance relationship, but there are many alternatives to meeting in person: a video call over Skype, sending messages on social media, even an email exchange. What do you even talk about when you meet up? Whatever it is that human beings talk about. Talk about your favorite movies, the places you grew up, what you do for a living, how terrible the traffic was on the way here, or take the opportunity to lovingly make fun of the partner you share.

You may come out of this meeting with an awesome new friend, or you may feel decidedly "meh" about this person. You may have loads in common, or you may be polar opposites. At the bare minimum, this should establish an open channel of communication. At best, this makes it way easier to plan things like elaborate surprise parties for your partner in common, and also allows you to coordinate and communicate should your partner in common end up in some kind of emergency situation.

When You're the Partner in Common

When you are the partner in common between two people (the pivot point of a vee relationship), there are a few simple things you can do to encourage harmonious relationships between your metamours. It's best to avoid being the broker as much as possible. Brokering sets you up as the intermediary between your partners. Although at the very beginning you are the only link between these two (or more) individuals, it's best to encourage your metamours to create connections between themselves independently. No one likes to be the go-between, transmitting information between metamours in what inevitably becomes a frustrating game of telephone. If one of your partners takes issue with another, encourage him to confront your other partner directly. If there's an open channel of communication there, hashing out differences should not be a major problem.

Why Bother?

Why bother going through the effort of reaching out to your metamours? Why care whether or not your partners ever meet each other? It comes back to that need for cohesion in your tribe. Everyone needs to feel like they are on the same team. In order for any polyamorous relationship to work, your partners cannot see each other as rivals. Before meeting your metamour face-to-face, you may have envisioned your partner's other partner as your competition, as someone smarter and prettier than you, as a living embodiment of your partner's desire for someone who doesn't have all your flaws. When you meet your metamour, it gives you a chance to see her as a human being, stripped away of all the crud your brain has attached to her. You have the opportunity to get to know a person who wants the same things that you do: to feel safe, to feel wanted, to love freely, to be happy. Create an environment where your metamour can get all of those things, and it's likely you'll find that she will do the same for you.

Cohabiting

Part of creating your tribe may involve sharing living space with someone you love (or multiple people that you love). Cohabiting or "nesting" comes with both benefits and difficulties, and it's firmly established as one of the steps on the relationship escalator (usually as a precursor to getting married). Society at large expects that any serious relationship will eventually lead to cohabitation, but this may not be realistic or beneficial for all relationships. Take some time to examine what you really want. You may see yourself able to live with certain partners, but never with others. Or you may be much happier living with someone who doesn't have any romantic or sexual ties, such as a friend or a family member. You may welcome the idea of sharing space with multiple partners and your meta-mours, or you may prefer to live solo. Either way, don't let expectations of the relationship escalator get in your way. You may have a passionate relationship that lasts decades without ever cohabiting, or you may find yourself happily moving in with a chosen family of partners and metamours.

If you are considering moving in with one or multiple romantic partners, here are a few things to keep in mind. This is far from a comprehensive list, and they are not listed in a particular order. For much more specific information and guidance on the logistics of polyamorous cohabitation, check out *The Polyamorous Home* by Jessica Burde.

- *Discuss the environment you want.*
Before moving in, have frank conversations about the kind of environment you need to feel comfortable at home. Does the entire place need to be sparkling clean at all times? Or do you just need to have a personal space that is tidy? What are your expectations about the noise level of music, movies, etc.?

- *Be sure that everyone has access to personal space.*
If you are a couple moving in together, chances are you are planning on sharing a bedroom. After all, looking for a one-bedroom place saves so much on rent! However, what you save in rent may not make up for the frustration that comes later on when neither of you feel like you can escape each other. A good guideline is to seek out a place that has the same amount of space that you would want if you were moving in with a roommate and not a lover. It doesn't mean that you won't share a bedroom, but it does mean that you'll have room to get out of each

other's hair when necessary. If you are moving in solely for financial reasons, this may be a lot harder to do.

If you are moving in with multiple partners, you need to discuss sleeping arrangements. Does everyone get their own bedroom? Does everyone sleep together in the same bed?

• **Discuss how you will schedule dates and sleepovers with others.**

The person you choose to live with will immediately become privy to your comings and goings. This means that the logistics of scheduling nights out or sleepovers with other partners will require thorough communication. If you go out on a date and spend the night with someone, out of courtesy you'll have to let your partner back at home know that you won't be coming back that night. If you want a partner to come stay the night at your place, you and your nesting partner may have to compare schedules to find a night when he may be off having his own sleepover with one of his other partners. In time, this kind of communication becomes par for the course. If you are currently in the habit of not updating your partner when you're planning a date, expect that there may be an adjustment period as you start keeping him up-to-date on your calendar.

• **Share a calendar.**

Because scheduling multiple partners' time can become a tangle very quickly, it can be helpful to share a calendar with one or several of your partners. Instead of needing to get the weekly rundown, you can see at a glance when your partner has plans or prior commitments. There are plenty of mobile and browser-based apps that allow you to exchange calendars with other people. Bear in mind that sharing a calendar may not always be appropriate, depending on the intensity of the relationship and the comfort level of the people involved. Some people prefer relying on open communication rather than being able to see their partners' every move at all times.

• **Talk about the bed.**

The bed you sleep in every night takes on an odd sense of the sacred. Some couples who are newly opening their relationship create agreements surrounding the bed they share. These might include strictly forbidding each other from bringing anyone new into their home at all, or it may simply be an agreement to change the sheets after any sexual activity (it's nice to save your partner from that ick factor). For the sake of logistics, being okay with sleeping in other people's beds and being okay with other people sleeping in yours makes things far easier. Treat another person's sleeping space with the same respect you would want someone to treat your own.

- **Not everyone will be on board.**

When you live with one or multiple partners, it becomes part of the information you must disclose to potential partners. And you may be dismayed to find that this scares people away . . . even other poly folk! Some people see cohabiting as a sign of relationship importance and life entwinement (and usually it is), but may think this means that you will not have any more room in your life for a new partner, physically or emotionally. If you genuinely do not have that space for a new partner, you must be honest with yourself and others about that. If not, take extra care to communicate your other relationship commitments honestly, but assure new partners that you are willing to dedicate time, energy, and effort to new relationships as well.

- **Your partners will have to meet each other (and you'll have to meet your metamours).**

If you are used to keeping your relationships compartmentalized, with little interaction between your partners and metamours, that's about to change. Or at least, it *should* change if you want to maintain your sanity.

"Hey, come over to my place tonight! But it has to be after 7 p.m. because my husband is here until 6:30, and you have to be out of here before he gets back at 10 p.m. But he might get back earlier. He'll text me when he's heading back, so when he texts me we have to drop whatever you're doing and get out of here because if we are all in the same room together at the same time someone's head might explode."

It's a logistical nightmare that sounds ridiculous here, but is reality for many non-monogamous couples who choose to cohabit. Better to make friends with your metamours ahead of time, and make the effort to introduce your partners to each other. It doesn't mean that anyone automatically gets to move in or disrespect your private space, but it means that everyone can be in the same room at the same time without the threat of head explosion.

- **A logistical hierarchy may develop.**

Whether you subscribe to established relationship hierarchy or not, cohabiting will establish a sort of logistical hierarchy into your love life. The partner(s) that you live with will generally need to be kept abreast of when you're going out on dates, whether or not you'll be spending the night elsewhere, and who you might be bringing home.

Spontaneous interactions with your partners will require more mindfulness as well. If you and your cohabiting partners are binge-watching on the couch in your pajamas, and you receive a text inviting you to go down the road and grab a drink with your other partner who happens to be in the neighborhood, what do you do? If you were living by yourself, you could clean yourself up and head out the door without a second thought. But now that you're living with someone, you have to consider whether or not she might feel hurt by your bailing in the middle of your time together. This isn't to say that spontaneous get-togethers are off the table, but they will require more communication with your nesting partner.

- *Plan for some separation.*

When you live with a partner, usually you'll find yourself spending far more time with this person than you would otherwise. This is someone (or multiple someones) you'll wake up with every morning, go to bed with every night, and collaborate with on "adulting"—managing household bills, washing the dishes, doing the laundry, etc. This is important time that will deepen your bond, but it can also lead to a loss of excitement and attraction.

It's important to maintain some separation in your relationship in order to sustain attraction. If you and your living partner are free to seek your own interests, pursuits, and relationships, it injects the breathing space necessary to keep things from getting dull. If you are still creating a life independent from your partner, you are still growing, changing, learning, and being an interesting human being for your partner to continue to discover!

- *Don't let sex fall to the bottom of the list.*

If sex is an important part of your romantic relationship, bear in mind all that adulting can get in the way of maintaining a healthy, exciting sex life with your cohabiting partner. Many people report that having sex with a variety of partners actually contributes to their sex drive and sexual exploration within each relationship. After all, when you allow yourself to have multiple teachers, you learn a lot of cool tricks!

Still, some well-meaning people will spend most of their time focused on either work, family, household chores, or hobbies, then find they have no energy left for sex at the end of the day. The spirit may be willing, but the body is weak. Find a way to extend foreplay throughout the day (flirty text messages and sexy pictures work great for this). If you can, make time for sex to happen earlier in the day, rather than hoping that the day leaves enough time left over for sex to happen.

Kids in Poly Families

Dissenters of polyamory sometimes point out, "Yeah, that might be fun for now. But once you want to have kids it will be a different story." It certainly is a different story, but many people don't simply choose to stop being poly once they are ready to bring children into the world. In her book *The Polyamorists Next Door,* Dr. Elisabeth Sheff compiled fifteen years' worth of research on polyamorous family structures and the benefits and disadvantages of raising children within a poly household. Sheff found that children raised by not only their parents, but their parents' partners as well, enjoyed having the attention and care of multiple adults and felt confident and safe in their family's love. The biggest drawbacks that Sheff found were the difficulties the families encountered in combating stigma, sometimes directed at children far too young to handle a conversation with someone criticizing their parents' relationship choices.[1]

The most successful poly families with kids have a strong foundation of open, honest communication about relationships and sexuality. Though many parents choose to remain in the closet to protect their children from stigma, more poly families are beginning to share their voices.

"I am completely open with [my daughter] about the fact that I have multiple relationships. While I don't share intimate details of my sex life (that would be abuse!), she knows that non-monogamy is my relationship style and that when my partners come to visit, we sleep in the same bed. Just like monogamous people, when I have a new partner, I wait until I feel this person will add value to her life before introducing her. I'm out as poly in my community and feel that I have nothing to hide. My primary relationship with her other parent is same-sex so we have always had something a little different than those of her friends' families . . . Honesty is so important in our family! She has always appreciated the fact that we came out to her and that we always include her in conversations about partners visiting and family time, etc. She now has more loving adults around and sees that we are living in our truth and choosing to love in ways that align with our truest selves, even if it's not the same as the overall culture. Everybody wins!***"* —Paige

“Having a daughter has made me more aware that it's really important for me to know exactly what I want out of my sexual/romantic/love relationships. The better I know myself, the clearer and more effective I can be as a parent. Everything I do affects my daughter whether I like it or not, so I have that awareness . . . It is case by case when/if/how I introduce a lover/partner/boyfriend/girlfriend to my daughter. I tell her that she is number one and that no one is going to steal me away from her (she has voiced this fear). I try to show her that I only bring positive, inspirational people into our lives. We talk about sex but not about my love life or the fact that I am having sex because I think she's still too young. I tell her that we don't have a traditional mommy/daddy/daughter home and that it's okay. I tell her that she is free to make her own choices when she is an adult, and that she doesn't have to choose the way I chose. I tell her that it's important to be your authentic self and be comfortable with who you are even if it's different from others.**”**—Erica

An Interlude on Community

There is a massive house in Santa Monica affectionately and ironically known as The Church. The place has six bedrooms, three bathrooms, a craft room, a hot tub, a wall of Nerf weapons, a massive projection screen, a climbing wall, and an adult-sized ball pit in the backyard. There are events every single weekend, ranging from quiet movie nights to elaborate costume parties and fully organized Nerf-gun battles with established teams and sponsors. The house has hosted nerds and outcasts from all walks of life—nine-to-fivers and freelancers, lawyers, video game developers, artists, and the perpetually unemployed. It has been the stage for going-away parties, memorial services, *Magic: The Gathering* tournaments, and the occasional orgy.

The people who live at The Church, as well as those who frequent the place, are a healthy mix of polyamorous and monogamous, kinky and vanilla. When I was still living in Southern California, The Church came to be the physical hub of my little tribe of lovers, metamours, and friends. If I was dating someone new, it wouldn't be long before they would be brought to The Church to meet everyone else.

I had been seeing Jake for three or four weeks when I invited him to The Church to meet my partners Jase and Emily, who would be there with some of their other partners as well. I was giddy with excitement and nervousness.

My nerves turned out to be unfounded, because Jake instantly hit it off with everyone there. After sharing drinks and discussion in the kitchen, it was time to move on to my very favorite Church tradition: skinny dipping in the hot tub. Jase turned to Jake and said, "Jake, it's been wonderful to meet you. Now please take off your clothes."

Jake dropped his pants without a moment's hesitation, and we all relocated into the hot tub. If this were a steamy erotic novel, this would inevitably be the point where we all melted into a writhing orgy. In reality, it was like any other night naked hot tubbing at the Church: comfortably casual and likely boring to most onlookers.

I cuddled with Emily in the corner before watching her sidle over to her new boyfriend Josh. I floated between Jase and Jake for cuddles. Jase's other partner, Brooke, sat on the edge of the tub next to her boyfriend, Johnny. Brooke was particularly vigilant about delivering a vicious but playful smack on the ass to anyone who made the mistake of exposing themselves. Occasionally, people from inside the house would pop outside, pulling up a chair next to the hot tub to join the conversation for a while. We stayed there for a number of hours, discussing movies, travel, languages, video games, and any other number of topics.

This night stands out to me because of the way it made me feel. I felt happy within my small tribe—I was safe and cared for, surrounded by people who knew me and who were all on the same team. It felt so far removed from the world of managing jealousy, of negotiating boundaries and agreements and rules, of quelling feelings of insecurity or competitiveness. It just felt natural, comfortable, peaceful.

Within this particular group of people, inevitably there was change. Some relationships escalated, others de-escalated, some ended entirely. New connections were made, and new people were brought in. But regardless of the ebb and flow, I still aspire to this standard in my romantic life. I still aim for that sense of family, of community, of tribe. People and relationships shift and change, but that sense of cohesion and safety is precious and lasting.

"We have a custom-made family. I'm fortunate that my partner Louis and my partner Scott get along. When Louis's car broke down, he and Scott were able to fix it. Saved us lots of money. Scott's car broke down and Louis was able to loan him his. I guess the best memory is when we all had dinner together. I could tell Scott was a bit nervous *but Louis did his best to make him feel comfortable. We try to have dinner together about once every couple months. This is our way of checking in together.* **"** —Kara

"We are finding now that getting adequate family time, time with one another, and time with our partners is like piecing together a puzzle. My favorite moments are when everyone is in the same place at the same time, sharing a meal or spending time outside chatting all together. That's when my heart feels like it's going to shine through my whole body. It's wonderful.* **"** —Willow

Chapter 10 Homework

Exercise #1

If you were to build your tribe from scratch, who would it include? Make a list of at least five ideal people you would want in your community. This may include romantic partners, close friends, your partner's partners, or mentors. These people may already be in your life, or they may have yet to enter your life. If the latter, brainstorm where you might meet these people.

Exercise #2

Take stock of the relationships that you have with your metamours, whether brand-new or long established. Is there anything holding you back from creating a closer relationship with your metamours? Is there a history of conflict or tension? What are the ways in which you could create more cohesion in these relationships?

11 Polyamory: The Next Frontier

One day as I was clicking through my online news feed, I ended up on a conservative Christian blog that shared news stories that supported Biblical prophecies of an impending global apocalypse. I was sucked in by warnings of a coming economic collapse, tales of natural disasters around the world, and the horrors of church groups accepting an openly gay pastor. Not my usual reading material, but I was down the rabbit hole. I couldn't help but click the headline "Universities Across America Look to Mainstream Polyamory." The article was a simple roundup of pro-polyamory events and workshops being held on college campuses. It was surprisingly unbiased, and had no commentary or editorial interpretation save for the reference tag at the end of the article: DAYS OF LOT.

This a reference to the Biblical figure of Lot, who gathered up his family and valiantly escaped from Sodom and Gomorrah, two towns that were slated for divine destruction. There's debate as to what exactly these two towns did to get on God's hit list, but it's generally believed that it had to do with the townspeople engaging in some form of kinky sex. The Abrahamic God is not known for being the most sex-positive guy.

Polyamory entering mainstream awareness; transgender people battling for recognition and protection; the legalization of homosexual marriage. To the religious right, these are the signs of the end times, and divine retribution is just around the corner. To the liberal left, it's quite the opposite. These are victories, triumphs over the forces that would seek to shame and to silence. To others, these are the harbingers of a new era of acceptance, love, tolerance, and enlightenment. Regardless of which extreme you speak to, everyone seems to agree that we are living on the edge of change. Big shifts are happening. Either the world is going to hell in a handbasket, or we're entering the Age of Aquarius. Cue the song from *Hair*.

It's a dubious claim that more people embracing non-monogamous relationships is a sign that an apocalyptic catastrophe is on the horizon, but it's also not necessarily an indicator of our species' collective emotional and sexual transcendence. Culture is indeed changing, but what both the alarmists and the hopeful optimists fail to realize is that it has always been changing. That's the nature of existence. Whether said change is good or bad is relative. The only thing that's consistent is that change is going to happen regardless.

It's difficult to predict what the polyamory scene may look like five years, ten years, or fifty years from now. Freedom of gender identity, sexuality, and relationship choice are still intertwined and governed by political and religious authorities in many parts of the world, disenfranchising many who fall outside the boundaries of cisgender, monogamous heterosexuality. It is impossible to give full coverage to every issue relating to relationship, gender, and sexuality, but here is a brief snapshot of what's going on in the world at the time of this writing:

- **Gay Rights**

It is still possible to be imprisoned or put to death for being bisexual or homo-sexual in certain parts of the world, including many countries in Africa and the Middle East. Some countries that outlaw same-sex relationships specifically tar-get sex between men, turning a blind eye to lesbian relationships. Many countries recognize same-sex relationships, but do not grant rights equivalent to hetero-sexual marriage. However, gay rights extend beyond just marriage or official rec-ognition of union: these rights include equal access to healthcare, adoption and parenting resources, protection from discrimination and hate crimes, and many other basic civil rights.

Over the past forty years, gays and lesbians living in the United States have slowly gained more access to these rights. It wasn't until June of 2015 that the United States Supreme Court nationally legalized gay marriage, after decades of back and forth, heated debate, and rights granted and taken away by indi-vidual state legislations. Unfortunately, the issue is far from settled. The topic is still a subject of heated debate, and non-heterosexual people are still victims of hate crime and discrimination.

- **Transgender Rights**

Transgender people, long virtually invisible within the mainstream, have become a household conversation. Around the world, many countries are beginning to grant basic rights and recognition to individuals who identify as transgender or outside the male-female gender binary, including Ireland, Pakistan, India, Colombia, and Argentina, just to name a few.[1] The United States still has some catching up to do. Openly transgender people are barred from serving in the military, excluded by some health insurance companies, and have historically been victims of brutal hate crimes.

At the time of this writing, American media is awash in coverage of controversial "bathroom bills." These pieces of legislation vary from state to state, either granting transgender people the right to use the restroom of whichever gender they identify with or barring them from doing so, indicating that everyone must use whichever restroom matches the sex listed on one's birth certificate. Ironically, transgender people have been using whichever restroom they please for decades now without much hubbub, and the transgender community argues that it should stay that way. Dissenters claim that this would make it easier for dastardly men to enter women's restrooms and assault helpless ladies and little girls.

This current controversy points to an issue far larger than just toilets. For many, this stands as a desperate attempt to keep the transgender community invisible and disregarded. This represents endeavors to maintain the status quo and keep everyone inside the "normalcy" of being cisgender and heterosexual. It seeks to uphold traditional gender roles and worn-out ideals of masculinity and femininity. It continues the process of "othering" those who fall outside traditional norms of sexuality and expression. It is no coincidence that this became the new hot-button issue not long after gay marriage was legalized. The outcome of these individual bathroom bills may show how much of a stronghold the religious right still has on the social development of the United States.

In May of 2016, the Obama administration administered a directive to public schools that offered guidance and suggestions for best practices in creating nondiscriminatory environments for transgender children and teenagers. The directive drew massive conservative backlash, as it held the veiled threat that federal funding would be pulled from schools that do not comply with the stated guidelines. Many business owners are boycotting the states that seek to restrict transgender rights, but dissenters still stubbornly fight for these pieces of legislation.

• *Women's Rights*
The history and present-day status of women's rights around the globe is a topic too broad to capture in a few paragraphs. Within the United States, the last one hundred years has seen the birth of women's suffrage, legal protections against discrimination, and increasing access to birth control and reproductive care.

However, the stability of some of these rights (such as fair and equal pay, medical coverage for birth control, and access to legal, safe abortions) grow shaky and unreliable with shifting political tides and constant changes in policy.

Across the globe, women still suffer from egregious human rights violations. Some of these violations are endemic within a particular culture, such as female infanticide, genital mutilation, forced marriage, and honor killings. Others are more widespread, including domestic violence, employment discrimination, lack of property and inheritance rights, sexual harassment and assault in public and in private, limited access to proper healthcare, and a dearth of educational and career opportunities.

Despite the widespread prevelance and growing awareness of these issues, women continue to be underrepresented within the global political sphere. Only two countries in the world have 50 percent or more women sitting in their national parliament. The rest of the world averages a female parliamentary representation of approximately 23 percent.[2]

- ### *Human Rights and Intersectionality*

Your relationship choice may be criticized, vilified, or directly attacked on the basis of your sex, gender identity, or sexuality, but these are far from the only factors that may affect the degree of difficulty you might experience as you seek any number of basic human rights. For this reason, it is important to look at all of these issues, including those facing the polyamorous community, through the lens of *intersectionality*.

Intersectionality begins with recognizing that every person may own multiple identities (e.g. you may identify not only as a woman, but as a woman of color, a parent, a lesbian, and a survivor of abuse). These multiple identities can result in very different experiences for the person in question, regarding how they experience discrimination. It can be tempting to see intersectionality as a numbers game—a way to one-up others in a race to see who is more victimized and who is more privileged. However, it's imperative to realize that intersectionality merely points to the fact that each human being's experience of privilege and discrimination will be different based on the unique qualities of their multiple identities, rather than just the quantity of identities.

Your privileges and disadvantages in the arena of relationships, sex, and other areas of life may be different based on your race, skin color, level of education, socioeconomic status, ethnic background, religion, disability, income level, age, country of origin, mental or physical health, living situation, or any other number of unique factors.[3]

How Does Polyamory Fit Into This?

The communities mentioned face unique challenges that are distinct from those faced by the polyamorous community. However, what's held in common is the entanglement of personal freedoms with government regulation, the clash of traditional ideals with progressive thinking, the struggle to protect the wholesome normal folk from all the deviant weirdos. It goes beyond the fear of someone who looks, talks, acts, and lives differently from the norm. The long-standing rhetoric has been that traditional family values are under attack from all sides: by the so-called gay agenda, by the feminist movement, by transgender individuals, and now by the non-monogamous.

One of the main reasons that these movements are perceived as threatening is because they fundamentally challenge long-held views on sex. The belief that sex should be only for the purposes of procreation is a driving force behind maintaining a rigidly gender-divided and sex-negative culture. To recognize things such as homosexual attraction and love, the desire for multiple partners, or the fluidity of gender itself is to acknowledge that sex is more than just body parts and reproduction. To take off the blinders and see the sexuality that happens outside the box of heteronormativity is to see the full spectrum of what sex is for human beings. So much more than propagation, sex is part of our personal expression, a way to bond with others, and, if it's all going well, extremely pleasurable. For hundreds of years, the Puritan undercurrent in American culture has taken major issue with pleasure. There's a collective neurosis surrounding pleasure, and it is fundamentally believed that pleasure cannot be had for pleasure's sake. Instead, it must either serve some kind of purpose (such as producing children) or be earned through some amount of suffering (no cupcake until you've done your time in the gym that day). To indulge in pleasure for its own sake, especially sexual pleasure, is still a basis for condemnation and judgment. From the outside, having multiple partners appears shamelessly indulgent, and polyamorists in particular are often criticized as being selfish. As critics of poly often say, you can't have your cake and eat it too.

Dr. Elisabeth Sheff coined the phrase "fear of the polyamorous possibility." Once a person becomes aware of the possibility of openly maintaining romantic and sexual relationships with multiple partners, there's a potential for extreme reactions of disdain, disgust, and fear. Women in the poly community have shared tales with me of monogamous female friends suddenly keeping a tighter grip on their husbands and boyfriends after learning that someone they know is practicing polyamory. Well-meaning friends have reached out to me saying, "I want to give your Facebook page a 'like,' but if my girlfriend saw what your podcast was about, she would murder me." A work colleague looked over my website once and started to ask me questions about polyamory before suddenly stopping short and saying, "I want to ask more questions, but if I go down the rabbit hole then there won't be any going back. For the sake of my marriage, let's stop talking about it." Like much homophobic rhetoric, there is an inherent fear that there is some force of licentious deviancy that is trying to convert and corrupt the virtuous.

Sheff argues that this fear is so common because nearly everyone can relate to some part of non-monogamy,[4] either through experiencing or acting on a desire for someone who is not their current partner, or being aware and fearful that their partner might feel that same desire for someone else. To be presented not only with the possibility of non-monogamy, but also the idea that it could be a viable, healthy option, is challenging to many people. To some, the poly-amorous possibility represents chaos, a loss of control, and the threat of losing a partner to someone else. Some see an implicit attack on traditional marriage, monogamy, and the nuclear family unit. Surely the very foundations of society would crumble if everyone got to have their cake and eat it too. At the very least, we'd be all out of cake in no time.

Those who decry the purported war on traditional family values make the mistake of looking at the concept of family as just that: a tradition. Getting presents from your parents on every night of Hanukkah is a tradition. Counting down to midnight on New Year's Eve is a tradition. These are customs that have been passed down from generation to generation. Some traditions survive because they maintain their original significance, and some survive through unquestioned repetition long after their origins have been obscured by time.

Family, however, goes beyond tradition or customs. The current "tradition" of family may look fairly cookie cutter: mommy, daddy, and two-point-five kids. Family is so much more expansive than this. Like the chosen family or the tribe mentioned in chapter 10, the expansive family is a fundamental truth of our human nature. This is the family that cannot come under attack from anything, because it can be found regardless of circumstances, location, or legislation. This is the family that we choose individually, populating it with people who enrich our lives and hold us up through the difficulties of existence. To choose this family or tribe, whether it be through marriage, adoption, cohabiting, or everyday association, is our birthright as human beings.

Critics claim that these movements seek to destroy tradition and the conventional family, but it may be more accurate to say that these movements seek to widen the spectrum of acceptance. This includes the polycule of lovers and partners living together becoming just as acceptable as the standard two-parent home with a white picket fence. It includes the transgender man walking into the men's restroom without fear of harassment, just as a cisgender man can. It includes a man's pursuit of paternity leave being just as admissible as a woman taking maternity leave. Widening the range of acceptance and understanding also widens the possibility for happiness and peace on a societal level.

Non-Monogamous Marriage Rights

Long before the Supreme Court's decision, conservatives had argued that if gays were allowed to marry, it would soon be a slippery slope to people being allowed to marry children, animals, or even multiple people at the same time! In the wake of the legalization of gay marriage, there was an immediate uproar from the conservative media, warning that it would only be a matter of time before we are a society of bestial, bigamist pedophiles. Alarmists pointed to tragic cases of child-brides forced into group marriages with deranged cult leaders, and wealthy Middle Eastern aristocrats collecting massive harems of wives and mistresses.

Others in the media were quick to counter these arguments—it's ridiculous to assume that it would ever be legal for someone to marry an entity that could not give consent (namely a child or an animal). However, this also meant a surprising backlash against non-monogamy from the liberal media, which historically has shown more hesitant curiosity than outright hostility toward the subject. Numerous news outlets ran op-eds assuring that gay marriage would not lead to multi-partner marriage, because there's no way *that* kind of relationship could ever work in the first place.

The polyamorous community finds itself in a strange position. There has yet to be a strong call to advocate for marriage rights for the non-monogamous. Most people who are willing to step outside the boundaries of traditional relationship rules have also abandoned any conviction about the institution of marriage, yet the lack of formal recognition has allowed job and housing discrimination, child custody battles, and long-standing relationships barred from partaking of the benefits currently granted to married couples.

There has yet to be a recognized ringleader campaigning for non-monogamous marriage rights, mostly because the community is still divisive on this subject. Those who do want multi-partner marriage have yet to make a decisive plan for how that could be effectively implemented. Some call for the expansion of marriage to include more than one person, allowing for triad or group marriage. This would require multiple people to be part of the same marriage contract, which would likely lead to logistical nightmares should anyone want to divorce. Other multi-partner marriage advocates claim that allowing overlapping dyadic (two-person) marriages would be more realistic. This means that in a triad relationship, there would be a total of three separate yet simultaneous marriages, rather than one group marriage. If one person wanted to leave the triad, it would involve negotiation between each individual dyad. The process would still be complicated, but would be better able to mirror existing laws surrounding divorce and property.

Still others in the community would rather advocate for shifting our cultural view away from seeing marriage itself as the all-important foundation of family and society. For this, we would need to focus on increasing the rights of those who are not interested or able to enter into a standard marriage contract. This would involve allowing single people to receive benefits normally reserved only for married couples, such as tax breaks and reductions in health insurance costs and university tuition. It's also necessary to consider the rights of people who wish to raise children without entering a dyadic marriage to do so.

With a lack of formal protection or recognition, some poly folk have turned to the infrastructure of business partnerships. The business world has many more options for handling contracts and supporting entities composed of multiple people, such as LLCs and Subchapter-S corporations. In the future, marriage contracts may be able to become similarly manifold in order to support a wide variety of relationship formats.

Whatever the outcome, it is becoming increasingly apparent that non-monogamous individuals require some type of formal recognition. This may be in the form of sanctioned marriage or domestic partnership rights, or in legal protections against relationship choice discrimination in housing or the workplace. The road to legal recognition has historically proven to be a difficult one, and widespread acceptance may fluctuate depending on the shifting political climate. The polyamory movement has its own obstacles to tackle, but the path has already been paved by the sacrifices made by those fighting for the rights of women and the LGBTQ community.

Parenting Rights

Legal recognition of multi-partner relationships may come not in the form of marriage rights, but parenting rights. Poly researcher Dr. Elisabeth Sheff suggests that it may be necessary for society to shift its perspectives on family from being based in marriage to being based on children and parenting.[5] Not all poly folk seek to raise children, but for those that do, advocating for shared parenting rights may be the fastest road to recognition and protection. At the time of this writing, California is the only state that has changed legislative standards to allow a child to have more than two legally recognized parents.[6]

Feminism

The feminism movement has seen many different evolutions since its inception. Granting women equal rights and the privilege of being seen as wholly human has been the through-line of feminism. The right to vote, own property, seek employment, and hold a driver's license, among many other rights, are still not guaranteed for women across the globe. The modern feminist movement still seeks to solidify equal pay, abortion rights, and social autonomy, and to combat many other destructive forms of sexism.

How does polyamory align with feminist ideology? Some old-school feminists decry non-monogamy, claiming that the modern-day movement is merely the oppressive, patriarchal polygamy of old stuffed into a hip and trendy re-packaging. An extreme assumption, but understandable. Witnessing a woman in a relationship with a man who is enjoying multiple other women at the same time can trigger those images of harems and cult leaders. But even in healthy non-monogamous, heterosexual relationships, does the sexual autonomy of the man inherently mean the woman is still suffering under the thumb of the patriarchy? As much as she claims to have actively chosen polyamory, is she really, deep down, just doing it to please her man? (Note: non-monogamous gay and lesbian relationships do not seem to trigger the same outcries from doubting feminists.)

Feminists in support of non-monogamy point to the ideally equal-opportunity nature of effective non-monogamous relationships. Unlike the controlling polygamy of the past, polyamorous women are more likely to have equal access and opportunity to pursue multiple partners. For this to work, not only does the woman herself need to feel empowered enough to feel free and happy to fulfill her various sexual and romantic desires, but her partners must have abandoned archaic beliefs about controlling female sexuality that are still firmly embedded in our social psyche at large. Anyone who still views a woman responsibly engaging with multiple partners as slutty, promiscuous, or any other pejorative is unlikely to want to be in a relationship with that woman in the first place.

Social environments that support a woman's sexual autonomy this completely are historically rare, which is perhaps why women frequently hold positions of authority and power in current non-monogamous circles. Statistically, more women than men request open relationships,[7] and the majority of books published on polyamory and non-monogamy have been written by women. Slightly more men than women identify as polyamorous,[8] meaning that hetero-sexual poly women have access to a greater variety of options when selecting male partners, quite contrary to the maligned imagery of harems and sister-wives.

Much of polyamorous rhetoric discourages competitiveness as well, which is antithetical to the social atmosphere at hand that often pits women against each other. The status quo of media and advertising keeps women constantly reminded that their greatest stronghold of power and value is in their beauty. This beauty is the foremost tool in acquiring the status of coupling with an influential man. It is the unspoken expectation that a woman's goal is to out-pretty every other woman around. On top of this, centuries of men being the only source of security for socially disempowered women has developed a collectively held bad habit of needing to defend your man from being stolen by another woman at all costs. But in an arena where no one can claim total ownership over their partner, it's difficult to justify a default of suspicion and rivalry toward other women.

Does this all add up to mean that polyamory is inherently feminist? It is difficult to give a definitive yes or no. The swinging community, established decades prior to the modern polyamory movement, still comes under similar scrutiny. Swingers espouse that women hold most of the power in the scene, enjoying the ability to seek out all manner of sexual fantasies and receive copious respect surrounding consent and boundaries. Yet critics point to the still common practice in swinging circles of a man approaching a woman's male partner first in order to be granted permission to play with her.

In a similar vein, polyamory is not by its very nature exempt from disempowering habits that carry over from a long-established history of patriarchy. The unfortunately frequent occurrence of One Penis Policy relationships in the polyamory scene smacks of male privilege and insecurity, as well as an innate undervaluing of female-female relationships. Previously monogamous couples who seek to add a third to their relationships often hunt down the fetishized fantasy of the hot bisexual woman—perfectly tailored to titillate the man without being threatening. (See chapter 8.)

Yet, for every gender-imbalanced non-monogamous relationship, there are even more in which both women and men are free to seek partners of whichever gender or sexual orientation they desire. Are there non-feminists who pursue and find happiness in poly relationships? Of course. But in my opinion, those who do identify as feminist are likely to have more fun with it.

Poly-defensive

The polyamory movement continues to see small victories of awareness and acceptance, but the struggle is far from over. Fortunately, there are a growing number of excellent role models for the poly community that are raising their voices, creating content, and leading the campaign for freedom of relationship choice. However, there is an unfortunate side effect of having to constantly present the best face of non-monogamy. In an ongoing push for polyamory to be seen as valid and normal, it is difficult to publicly acknowledge darker topics.

Acknowledging Abuse

It can be tempting to think that poly relationships are more likely to be healthy. For a non-monogamous relationship to be effective and happy, it does require a number of healthy habits, such as self-efficacy and communication (and others discussed in chapter 4). But like any relationship, even non-monogamous relationships can grow unhealthy and act as a backdrop for physical, mental, or emotional abuse.

Abuse is a difficult subject for many of us to talk about, regardless of the relationship context. It becomes even more tricky considering that not all abuse is as obtuse as it's portrayed in the movies: the raging man physically taking out his aggression on a helpless partner. Physical abuse in particular usually relies on isolation of the abused partner in order to continue. In poly relationships involving multiple people, it is more difficult to hide physical abuse or get others connected to the relationship to allow it to perpetuate.

Emotional and mental abuse arise in ways that are much subtler, more difficult to detect, and can be sustained in relationships for years. Because polyamorous relationships often require people to enter the intensely vulnerable process of negotiating for their needs, there is fertile ground for fear-motivated emotional manipulation, guilt, and power games. These are problems in any two-person relationship, and it can get particularly ugly when it reaches the level of a romantically involved group. Because there is already relatively low awareness of recognizing nonphysical abuse in relationships, it is even more challenging to discuss it within a polyamorous context. There is more discussion on recognizing abuse and the particular forms it can take in non-monogamous relationships in chapter 8.

Predators

A predator is someone who seeks to exploit others. Just as abuse can be difficult to recognize and label, knowing when someone is a predator is a tough call. The word itself is sensational, usually affixed to pedophiles and rapists. Not all predators are sexual in nature, but polyamory and other non-monogamous scenes present an appealing image to those who are seeking sexual exploits.

It's theorized that more men than women come to polyamory because it implies an opportunity to freely have sex with several women with little effort and no consequences. Polyamory activist and blogger Pepper Mint named this the "Valley of the Dolls" fantasy.[9] Books, movies, TV, and pornography have created the myth that somewhere out there is the kind of woman who is ready to have sex at any moment, no questions asked. This woman is the very embodiment of DTF, and it doesn't matter whether she is even attracted to the man in question. Even better, there may be a place out there where there are several of these women in the same place, already warmed up and more than willing to engage in the most titillating of a man's fantasies. If you think this sounds extreme, take a look at nearly any mainstream pornography.

Most adults can distinguish between fantasy and reality, but something strange happens when an individual who has been consistently exposed to this fantasy is introduced to polyamory. On the surface, it resembles some of the key elements of the Valley of the Dolls fantasy: this is a community where you're likely to encounter sexually liberated women who are supportive of a person having multiple sex partners. This alone is enough for many people, and predators, to say, "Sign me up!"

This little glimpse of fantasy is a gateway. A predator may assume that if a woman shows some sign of sex positivity, she may very well be ready to get it on right then and there. Many a poly woman has consistently complained that certain men, upon learning that she is non-monogamous, automatically interpret it to mean that she is happy to fuck whoever crosses her path, including him. Predators may feel that a sex-positive environment entitles him to sex. He will use a person's sex-positive nature to justify exploitative behavior, such as being pushy, aggressive, demanding, manipulative, or violating boundaries and consent. Keep in mind that these assumptions and behaviors may not be conscious. The predator may regularly be confident, charming, and generally likable, with little awareness of his own predatory energy.

One night I joined a group of friends and partners to attend a local poly meet-up group. The evening began with discussion circles, and then transitioned into a clothing-optional pool party (but emphasizing that this would not be any kind of play party). The night had been enjoyable, but the energy took a darker turn as the party began to wind down. Several men, most of them new to the poly scene, began cornering women, growing more pushy and aggressive. As I was leaving the pool, a guy I had been talking to through the evening asked me not to go several times, going so far as to roughly grab my arm and try to pull me back when I said no. The next day, as I was complaining to a friend about this, she responded with, "Well, you were at a naked poly pool party. What do you expect?"

Like abusers, predators are an issue in any community. But within more sexually liberated circles, it is difficult to raise complaints about predatory behavior within a wider context because of sentiments like these. Rape culture is still fueled by the idea that the onus of violation is on a woman's behavior: how she dresses, speaks, acts, or the environment she has chosen to be in. If a woman is already "asking for it" by dressing in a revealing manner, then it's easy to assume that she is practically begging for it by being in sex-positive environments, such as poly meet-ups or swingers' parties. There is an underlying perception that by entering such an environment in the first place, a woman has already given her consent to anything that may follow. She has set foot into the Valley of the Dolls, and there's no going back.

Confronting Predatory Behavior

Calling out predators is difficult, especially if the person in question is a respected member of their poly community. Public shaming can destroy cohesion and burn bridges. Gossiping behind someone's back, even in the interest of warning others, creates a hostile environment rife with politics and hearsay. Choosing to say nothing allows the problem to perpetuate.

If your poly community can come together to confront someone's predatory behavior with an approach of compassion and healing, then all power to you. If not, the responsibility may fall on you to confront a person on their predatory behavior when you witness it, again with the aim of guidance. Remember that this person may not even have an awareness of the mistakes they are making. However, if the predator in question continues the behavior, even after confrontation and discussion, it may be time to cut ties.

Underrepresented Groups

The public face of polyamory, once nonexistent, is beginning to develop as the movement gains more traction and media coverage. The going is slow, however, as the media flocks to cover the sensational and scandalous topic of non-monogamy in the safest and least offensive way possible. Journalists usually seek out white, heterosexual couples in an open relationship for interview subjects. It is rare that any partners outside of the couple are interviewed or even mentioned by name. Often there's a lot of focus on unicorn-hunting couples who are only seeking bisexual women to enhance the relationship. In other words, the media seeks to represent polyamory in a way that looks as close to monogamy as possible: couple-oriented and nonthreatening to men.

Though this media coverage provides a valuable source of exposure and awareness, it is hardly representative of the community at large. The movement has come under fire for appearing to be populated by the privileged: cisgender, white, middle- to upper-class, educated, and well-off enough to be able to hire a babysitter on date night and call a therapist whenever there's an emotional crisis. While there are many of these folks in the poly scene, these are also the people most likely to offer themselves up for media or research interviews. For this demographic, the potential consequences of being out of the closet and publicly visible are not insubstantial, but the stakes are significantly higher for members of other socio-economic and racial groups.

To openly identify as polyamorous is often out of the question for those whose identity is already subject to negative stereotypes. Those who are living with mental illness are vulnerable to having their unconventional relationships blamed on their condition, or being warned that their relationships may exacerbate their condition. Survivors of abuse invite the blame to be placed on them for engaging in a "deviant" relationship in the first place. And minorities are already wading through hackneyed and fetishized stereotypes about their sexuality: black women are freaky, Latin women are passionate, Asian women are submissive.

Black women and other women of color in particular have encountered certain difficulties participating in the poly community. Storyteller and poly activist Daniela Capistrano shares her thoughts on the ways in which institutionalized racism and privilege have affected her own poly relationships:

“*As a non-black, queer woman of color with light-skinned privilege, it's my responsibility to unpack and be accountable for the ways that anti-blackness has informed how I move in the world and how I've caused harm. It doesn't matter that I'm a person of color—this does not exempt me from looking at how racial dynamics play out in my relationships. To be a healthy poly person, it's my job to identify, accept, and heal how anti-blackness shows up in my behaviors and interpersonal dynamics. It is not my black partners' jobs to do this work for me. I've been fortunate that my poly life partner, Tracey Brown, who is a queer black woman and poly educator/speaker, has been very patient with me. But she shouldn't have to do this emotional labor. No black person should. It's MY job to be constantly vigilant and mindful of how my actions impact others in my poly relationships and how my priv-ileges, even as someone who experiences various forms of oppression, may sometimes blind me to the harm I'm causing.* **"**

The non-monogamous community is widespread and growing, though most people are only aware of the tip of the iceberg. The majority of the most pro-lific and publicly acknowledged writers within the poly community live up to the privileged image most often represented in the media: white, educated, and financially stable. There is a crucial need for the poly community to create a supportive and normalized space for a diverse range of voices and experiences.

Chapter 11 Homework

Exercise #1

How do you see yourself fitting into the future of the polyamory movement? Even if you don't choose to practice polyamory, do you see yourself continuing to support acceptance of relationship choice? What are the ways (big or small) that you can contribute to creating a positive environment for all relationship formats?

Conclusion: Going Within and Going Beyond

I am sitting in a cafe. Sitting across from me is my metamour, Jase's partner Reina. There are tears streaming down her cheeks. The night before, she had gone on a first date. She had only discovered polyamory when she met Jase a few months before. She had told her date about being polyamorous beforehand, and he had expressed interest and curiosity. However, the night turned sour when he began touching her and fondling her. They had both been drinking, and Reina, though uncomfortable with her date's advances, was inebriated enough that she didn't resist. It was only when he suddenly attempted to have unprotected sex with her that she had the presence of mind to call a halt to the action. Fortunately, her date stopped, and they parted ways. But Reina was still upset.

"I've been told my whole life to be nice and to not hurt a guy's feelings," she said. "I feel horrible about myself for not stopping him sooner. But I also feel horrible for even saying that I was polyamorous. Whenever I tell people that, they assume that I just want to have sex. How am I ever going to find good partners? How am I going to find people that love me?"

I was at a loss. I couldn't rush in and reassure her, *Oh, that guy was just a fluke. Shrug it off and move on to the next date.* I knew the harsh reality—that good partners *are* difficult to find, that being polyamorous *will* put you in the line of fire for every terrible sexual stereotype that's out there, and that by not conforming to traditional standards, she had signed up to play the dating game on "hard mode." But I also couldn't look her in the face and say, *Yeah, it sucks. Welcome to the life of a polyamorous woman.*

Why bother with this? I wondered. *Why go through the slog of looking for quality partners, letting go of jealousy, tackling uncomfortable self-work, awkwardly communicating your vulnerabilities, with no guarantee that any of it's going to work out?*

Then I remembered something that a meditation teacher had shared with me: *patience is the willingness to keep planting seeds, even if you don't know the hour when they will sprout.* Planting seeds requires getting dirty. You have to get on your knees, get dirt under your fingernails, get mud on your clothes. And there's no instant gratification. It requires putting in the uncomfortable work, even with the knowledge that you will not see results right away.

The pursuit of healthy relationships requires the same patience. This patience enables you to go within and confront your inner demons of insecurity, even though it's upsetting. It enables you to speak to your partner with kindness, even when your blood is boiling. It enables you to act with compassion and generosity, even when you feel jealous and competitive. It enables you to walk away from relationships that are not enhancing your life, even though it may be painful. Your patience frees you to let yourself get dirty, trusting that the results will manifest and unfold over time in healthy, balanced, fun, joyful, and deeply fulfilling relationships.

I shared this with Reina, grateful that her openness should inspire such a valuable reminder to myself, grateful that I could have a conversation and connection like this with a metamour. We talked more in depth about consent, dating culture, and relationships. She pulled up her Tinder profile, where she had wryly written: "Dislikes: People who think that poly women are easy."

As the conversation drew to a close, she looked at me, her eyes welling up again.

"Even after being in a relationship for eight and a half years, even after dating multiple people and having so many feelings, do I even know what love is?"

I had nothing for that one.

You may have asked yourself the same question, which has led you to go within yourself—to question everything about your relationships, your sex life, or your desires. That question may be what led you to this book, or it may have come up as you were reading this book. It certainly came up for me while writing it.

The more time I spend studying, experiencing, and experimenting with love, the more I find how much there is that I don't know. You may spend your entire life loving, and still only get a tiny sliver of understanding as to what the heck is actually going on. There are limitless, mysterious depths not only in love, but the myriad forms that relationships can take, the many facets of your partners, and the vast, shifting expanses within yourself. It may be impossible to get to the bottom of the depths within your own heart.

If there is anything you take away from this book, let it be this: keep planting those seeds, and keep exploring your inner depths over and over, with every new relationship and with every life milestone, with every moment spent quietly with one's thoughts. Continue a dogged pursuit of abandoning hand-me-down cultural assumptions and never cease to revisit the question, "What is love *to me*? What am *I* going to do about it?" The answer may always be a moving target, shifting and swaying and making sudden left turns as you shift and sway and make sudden left turns in your existence as a perpetually changing human being. The people in your life may not be able to hand you the answer, but love them from the depths of your soul, because each one gets you closer to it.

But let's take a step way back and look at the bigger picture as well. What does it mean that the polyamory movement should arise here, now? Is it just a passing fad among a bunch of millennials who have been scared out of commitment and monogamy by witnessing their parents' traumatic divorces? Are some of us striving to return to our basic human nature, abandoning modern definitions of love and family to get back to our non-monogamous roots? Or is it the dawning of a *new* New Age, a harbinger of a collective spiritual awakening and a renewed outpouring of love for all mankind? Will we eventually abandon monogamy altogether?

Both the people who feel threatened by the rise of non-monogamy and the people who feel inspired by it see it in the same way: as a radical force, capable of sweeping change. This change portents the end of a paradigm, a vehicle of destruction that would clear out our antiquated notions about family, marriage, love, and sex. It is seen as the end of monogamy, an event that is either delightful or horrifying, depending on who you talk to. This viewpoint paints polyamory as a *revolution*—an overthrow of the existing authority or status quo, potentially violent. Revolutionaries seek to replace the old school with something new, which is abjectly terrifying to those who are quite happy and comfortable with the old school. It is this alarm and fear of a revolutionizing force that gave rise to the rhetoric of the "gay agenda," which was steeped in the ridiculous fear that homosexuals seek to convert the straight and tear down the comfortable foundations of family life.

But even those who see a non-monogamous revolution as an unquestionably good thing have equally unreasonable beliefs. The narrative of the uplifting spiritual advancement of the human race depends on believing that we are making a mess of our inner selves as it is. It requires seeing monogamy as backwards and detrimental, and polyamory as a more enlightened and natural way of being. This portrays non-monogamy as not only a social revolution, but a spiritual one as well. But the polyamory movement is not about revolution. It's not about taking down the man, shaming the monogamous, disparaging vanilla sex, or vilifying traditional family life. Instead, this is about *evolution*.

Revolution is replacement, while evolution is expansion, transformation, and adaptation—*going beyond*. Evolution is universal and coexistent; all species gradually and uniquely adapt to meet the challenges of their individual environments. As species evolve, there are offshoots and exploratory mutations. Some carry on, and some fizzle out immediately. Some mutations serve a species perfectly until the environment changes. Drop a chimpanzee behind the wheel of a car, and you'll end up in a disaster. But if someone dropped you in the middle of the rainforest surrounded by hungry leopards, you'd find you're absolute rubbish at climbing the nearest tree and scurrying to safety. This doesn't mean chimpanzees are the superior species, nor does it mean that human beings are the superior species. It means that each are uniquely adapted to survive and thrive within their respective environments.

So it is with the blossoming awareness and acceptance of polyamory and non-monogamy. As a collection of human beings in different environments, with different needs, we are learning to adapt. We are shifting and adjusting to a world where every person can freely meet their romantic and sexual needs in a sustainable way, and that way may look different from person to person. We are building our acceptance for a variety of relationship formats, and creating a standard that allows for coexistence. I can get my needs met and find peace without needing to restrict someone else's ability to seek the same. Evolution isn't found in the polyamory movement itself, but in the fact that there is a growing space at all for polyamorists to exist, breathe, grow, and thrive. As more people become aware of that space, more people become aware that when it comes to relationships, there is a vast and unique world of variety, expression, practice, and choice. Between polyamory, swinging, relationship anarchy, or even consciously-chosen monogamy, there is a wide spectrum of relationship choice available to you. And having a choice, however limited or extensive, is the foundation of freedom.

Resources

There is a quickly growing world of information on alternative relationships. This list includes some of my favorite resources, though there are plenty more than mentioned here.

Books—Polyamory and Non-monogamy

More Than Two, Franklin Veaux and Eve Rickert (Thorntree Press, 2014). A comprehensive look at many aspects of modern polyamory, including solo and nonhierarchical polyamory.

Eight Things I Wish I'd Known About Polyamory: Before I Tried It and Frakked It Up, Cunning Minx (CreateSpace Independent Publishing Platform, 2014). An insightful examination of eight discoveries about consensual non-monogamy the author made in her first attempts at a poly relationship.

The Ethical Slut: A Practical Guide to Polyamory, Open Relationships & Other Adventures, Dossie Easton and Janet W. Hardy (Celestial Arts; 2nd edition, 2009). Long considered the "Bible" of polyamory, this classic book has seen many reprints.

The Jealousy Workbook: Exercises and Insights for Managing Open Relationships, Kathy Labriola (Greenery Press, 2013). Poly counselor Kathy Labriola presents exercises for systematically finding insights within jealousy, as well as determining relationship orientation.

Opening Up: A Guide to Creating and Sustaining Open Relationships, Tristan Taormino (Cleis Press, 2008). A thorough guide to a range of open relationship formats, though mainly written for couples looking to open up a closed relationship.

Polyamory: It's Not Complicated, DeWayne Lehman (CreateSpace Independent Publishing Platform, 2015). Irreverent, brash, and candid, Lehman shares his lessons learned from his time in the swinging and poly communities.

The Polyamorists Next Door: Inside Multiple-Partner Relationships and Families, Dr. Elisabeth Sheff (Rowman & Littlefield Publishers, 2013). After over a decade of research, Sheff presents her findings on the benefits and challenges faced by children raised in polyamorous households.

Polyamory in the 21st Century: Love and Intimacy with Multiple Partners, Deborah Anapol (Rowman & Littlefield Publishers, 2012). An analysis of modern-day polyamory mixed with historical research and personal anecdotes.

When Someone You Love Is Polyamorous: Understanding Poly People and Relationships, Dr. Elisabeth Sheff (Thorntree Press, 2016). A quick read designed to illuminate the basics of polyamory for friends and family members of people in polyamorous relationships.

The Polyamorous Home, Jess Mahler (Self Published, 2016). A thorough guide to maintaining poly-friendly living arrangements for a variety of relationship formats.

Books—Dating, Relationships, and Sex

If the Buddha Dated: A Handbook for Finding Love on a Spiritual Path, Charlotte Kasl (Penguin Books, 1999). A spiritual take on courtship and dating, though it is due for an update.

Sex at Dawn: How We Mate, Why We Stray, and What It Means for Modern Relationships, Christopher Ryan and Cacilda Jetha (Harper Perennial, 2010). This bestseller analyzes primate behavior and tribal cultures to make the case that human beings never evolved to be monogamous.

Good Sex: Getting Off Without Checking Out, Jessica Graham (Parallax Press, 2017). A frank and inclusive exploration of how mindfulness can make sex more connected, enlightening, and hot.

Sex From Scratch: Making Your Own Relationship Rules, Sarah Mirk (Microcosm Publishing, 2014). Nontraditional advice for dating and relationships with an emphasis on empowerment and autonomy to create unique relationships.

The New Topping Book, Dossie Easton and Janet W. Hardy (Greenery Press, 2011). A discussion of the rights and responsibilities of "tops," or those who have an interest in being sexually dominant.

The New Bottoming Book, Dossie Easton and Janet W. Hardy (Greenery Press, 2015). A discussion of the rights and responsibilities of "bottoms," or those who have an interest in being sexually submissive.

Books—Memoir

Wide Open: My Adventures in Polyamory, Open Marriage, and Loving on My Own Terms, Gracie X (New Harbinger Publications, 2015). An intimate account of the author's experiences opening her marriage and raising children with multiple partners in a polyamorous household.

The Game Changer: A Memoir of Disruptive Love, Franklin Veaux (Thorntree Press, 2015). A raw, vulnerable memoir detailing the author's destructive yet transformative eighteen-year open marriage.

My Life on the Swingset: Adventures in Swinging & Polyamory, Cooper S. Beckett (CreateSpace Independent Publishing Platform, 2015). Compiled from stories told on his popular blog and podcast, Beckett shares his lessons learned from years in the swinging community, which eventually led him to polyamory.

Stories From the Polycule: Real Life in Polyamorous Families, Ed. Dr. Elisabeth Sheff (Thorntree Press, 2015). An anthology of personal stories told by people in polyamorous families.

Books—Personal Development

The Untethered Soul: The Journey Beyond Yourself, Michael A. Singer (New Harbinger Publications/Noetic Books, 2007). An invaluable, life-changing book designed to bring mindfulness and awareness to the ways in which you speak and think about yourself.

The Art of Happiness, 10th Anniversary Edition: A Handbook for Living, Dalai Lama (Riverhead Books, 2009). A classic Socratic dialogue with the Dalai Lama on happiness and positive psychology.

5 Ways to Know Yourself: An Introduction to Basic Mindfulness, Shinzen Young (http://www.shinzen.org/). An accessible, logical manual for meditation and self-awareness.

The Fear Cure: Cultivating Courage as Medicine for the Body, Mind, and Soul, Lissa Rankin M.D. (Hay House, Inc., 2016). Dr. Lissa Rankin explains the ways that fear and stress compromise the body's immune system, and shows how our fears can be the gateway to our own healing.

Websites—Polyamory and Non-monogamy

Multiamory, *multiamory.com*. A wealth of information and advice for people interested in alternative relationships.

More Than Two, *morethantwo.com*. A comprehensive and long-running blog covering a wide variety of topics, accessible to both poly newbies and old hats.

Artichoke Love, *sirensongadultsalad.wordpress.com*. A blog written from the perspective of a pansexual, polyamorous woman on sex-positive parenting and non-monogamy.

Poly in the News, *polyinthemedia.blogspot.com*. A regular roundup of media coverage on polyamory.

Freaksexual, *freaksexual.com*. A blog written by queer and polyamorous activist Pepper Mint, with many excellent articles on men in non-monogamous circles.

Polyamory on Purpose, *polyamoryonpurpose.com*. A collection of practical advice for people in polyamorous relationships, with several articles on polyamory and mental illness and polyamory and pregnancy.

Loving More, *lovemore.com*. Originally one of the first print publications on polyamory; has now grown into an official nonprofit organization that holds regular events.

Frisky Fairy, *friskyfairy.com*. Dating coach and sex educator Rebecca Hiles writes on sex toys, creating a healthy sex life, and sex positivity.

Loving Without Boundaries, *lovingwithoutboundaries.com*. A blog on creating healthy, happy open relationships, featuring several interviews with other poly educators and authors.

Websites—Communication

The 5 Love Languages, *5lovelanguages.com*. A handy quiz for determining what your particular love language may be.

The Center for Nonviolent Communication, *cnvc.org*. Many free resources on nonviolent communication, as well as information on workshops and practice groups.

Dara Hoffman-Fox/Coming Out Worksheet, *darahoffmanfox.com/comingoutwork sheet*. Gender therapist Dara Hoffman-Fox offers one-on-one counseling and consultation for transgender individuals, as well as a handy worksheet for making a plan for coming out.

Websites—Online Dating

OkCupid, *okcupid.com*. This free dating network is currently the best option for those seeking polyamorous partners or alternative relationships, as it offers the widest range of profile filters for relationship orientation, sexuality, and gender identity.

OpenMinded, *openminded.com*. A site specifically marketed toward people looking for non-monogamous partners, though their approach is more couple-oriented.

Fetlife, *fetlife.com*. A massive online social network for people interested in kink.

Websites—Sexual Health

The following sites are the best places for up-to-date information on STI information and prevention, birth control, and overall sexual health.
Planned Parenthood, *plannedparenthood.com*.
World Health Organization, *who.int/topics/sexual_health*.
American Sexual Health Association, *ashasexualhealth.org*.

Centers for Disease Control and Prevention, *cdc.gov/sexualhealth*.

Podcasts

Multiamory, *multiamory.com/podcast*. A weekly podcast on non-monogamous relationships, sex, jealousy, boundaries, community, and much more.

Poly Weekly, *polyweekly.com*. One of the longest-running polyamory podcasts.

Life on the Swingset, *lifeontheswingset.com*. Covers the logistics of sexual and romantic exploration with an emphasis on openness and adventure!

Savage Love, *savagelovecast.com*. Dan Savage's classic radio show in podcast form, highlighting listeners' questions on love and sex.

Poly-friendly Coaches, Counselors, and Therapists

Kink-Aware Professionals Directory, *ncsfreedom.org/kap/*. The National Coalition for Sexual Freedom's directory of legal, medical, and therapeutic professionals who are aware or supportive of alternative relationships.

Dedeker Winston, *dedekerwinston.com*. My coaching services are available via Skype for singles, couples, triads, polycules, and more.

Cooper S. Beckett, *coopersbeckett.com/coaching*. Cooper brings years of experience in both swinging and polyamory to his one-on-one coaching.

Kathy Labriola, *kathylabriola.com*. Kathy is a licensed nurse and hypnotherapist with extensive experience working with people in non-monogamous relationships.

Sheffa Ariens, *sheffaariens.com*. Sheffa is a licensed marriage and family therapist who specializes in polyamorous, non-monogamous, and LGBTIQA clients.

Glossary

This glossary serves to clarify any specialized terminology used throughout the book. For a more comprehensive list of terms, I would recommend the More Than Two online glossary at *morethantwo.com/polyglossary.html*.

aromantic—a person who experiences very little to no romantic attraction to other people. May still experience sexual desire, but will often find satisfaction in friendships or other non-romantic interactions

asexual—a person who does not experience sexual attraction or strong desires for sex, but may still desire romantic and emotionally involved relationships

BDSM—BDSM is a combination of three different acronyms: Bondage/Discipline, Dominance/Submission, and Sadism/Masochism. It is often used as a catch-all term for any kind of power exchange, pain play, dominance, or other kinky play.

cisgender—used to describe a person whose gender identity matches their biological gender

compersion—a positive feeling of joy, excitement, and happiness when a loved one is feeling joy, excitement, or happiness about someone or something unrelated to you. Usually used to describe feeling happy when your partner has a good sexual or romantic experience with another partner.

cowboy/cowgirl—a derogatory term used to describe a monogamous person who dates a non-monogamous person with the intention of "taming" them and getting them to "settle down" with just one person

cuckold/cuckquean—a person who derives pleasure from their partner consensually "cheating" on them for a variety of reasons. The cuckold or cuckquean may get off from knowing that their partner is attractive and desired by others, or through eroticized feelings of humiliation. Cuckolds and cuckqueans may choose to take this fantasy outside of the realm of sexual play and allow their partner to pursue outside relationships.

demiromantic—also known as "gray romantic." A demiromantic person only experiences romantic attraction to a person after forming a close or familiar bond with them.

demisexual—a person who only experiences sexual attraction to a person after forming a close or familiar bond with them

D/s—Dominant and submissive. This abbreviation is used to describe a dominant and submissive relationship. The format of uppercase/lowercase is also used with other abbreviations that include a dominant and submissive component.

dyad—a relationship between two people. Can be used to describe a monogamous couple or a relationship between two people within a polyamorous network.

fluid bonding—an agreement between people who have chosen to have fully unprotected sex with each other, usually after STI testing and establishing reliable birth control. Some people choose to do this with only one person; some choose to do so with multiple people.

hetero-/homoflexible—a person who identifies primarily as heterosexual or as homosexual, yet under certain circumstances may choose to engage with members of whichever sex is outside of their usual preference

heteronormativity—the belief that all people fall into the categories of "male" or "female," that heterosexuality is the best (or only) acceptable relationship style, and that marriage and couple status are universal goals. It is also used to describe nontraditional relationships that try to look as similar as possible to traditional, heterosexual, long-term monogamy.

hierarchy—a relationship format that involves assigning specific partners as primary or secondary (and sometimes tertiary) to describe their level of priority. A hierarchy may involve rules or restrictions to ensure that the needs of primary relationship always comes first.

intersectionality—a theory and analytical tool for observing an individual's multiple identities and taking into account the wholly unique effect that individual's combination of identities may have on her access to human rights and experience of discrimination

kink—used to describe any nontraditional or nonconventional sexual practices including fetishes, paraphilias, role playing, and BDSM. The opposite of kink is *vanilla*, which is used for conventional sex.

metamour—your partner's other partners. Your boyfriend Josh's other girlfriend is Theresa. Theresa is your metamour.

monogamy—the practice of having only one romantic and sexual partner at a time

non-monogamy—any relationship structure that is not based on sexual or romantic exclusivity. A non-monogamous relationship may be consensual, such as swinging, cuckolding, or polyamory. Non-monogamy may also be non-consensual, as in infidelity or "cheating."

NRE—New Relationship Energy. The hormones and emotions that people experience when developing a new relationship. These chemical changes are very strong for the first few months and can last for over a year as they slowly revert back to normal levels.

NVC—Nonviolent Communication. A systematic method of conflict resolution wherein the communicator states an observation, shares their feelings, explains their needs, and then makes a request.

open relationship—a dyadic (two-person) relationship wherein each partner is free to pursue other partners sexually or romantically

OPP—One Penis Policy, a term used to describe a non-monogamous relationship where one or both members of a relationship are allowed to have sex with other women but not with other men

pansexual—a person who is sexually or romantically attracted to all gender identities. May also refer to a person whose sexual identity and attraction is fluid.

polyamory—engaging in multiple romantic relationships simultaneously with full knowledge and consent of all partners involved

polyandry—the practice of one woman having multiple husbands or male partners

polycule—a group of interconnected polyamorous relationships, including partners and metamours

polyfidelity—a closed relationship of more than two people who have agreed not to date or sleep with anyone outside of the polyfidelitous group

polygamy—the practice of having multiple spouses. In popular culture, this most frequently refers to a man who has multiple wives.

polygyny—the practice of one man having multiple wives or female partners

polysaturated—used to describe a polyamorous person who is not currently seeking new partners due to having their time and energy already occupied by other partners

relationship anarchy—a philosophy and practice of allowing all relationships to self-govern, without allowing external restrictions or cultural expectations to dictate the shape and agreements of each relationship. This may include eliminating the distinction between platonic and romantic relationships and allowing all relationships to take any form and have any level of commitment that the participants decide to have.

relationship escalator—used to describe the external cultural expectations put on a relationship to continue on a linear trajectory from dating to marriage to raising a family. This term is also used to describe the practice of treating a relationship as something that is moving toward a universal, external goal, such as cohabitation, marriage, or having children.

sex negativity—the belief that sex is inherently wrong, dirty, or immoral, and that sexual urges must be controlled or denied at all costs

sex positivity—the belief that sex, as long as it is healthy and consensual, is natural and positive

solo polyamory—a particular practice of polyamory that emphasizes an individual's own agency and independence, as opposed to creating a love life that is primarily couple-centric. These individuals may still have long-term committed relationships but may not seek to live with or share finances with a partner.

STI—a sexually transmitted infection

swinging—a practice where a couple may choose to engage in consensual sexual experiences with other people, usually with an emphasis on keeping any external relationship purely sexual and keeping romance exclusive to the couple. Some swingers may only sexually engage with others in certain contexts, such as at a play party, or they may have ongoing sexual friendships.

transgender—a person who self-identifies with a gender that is different from their biological sex. A transgender person may or may not have surgery or take hormones to change their external appearance, but it is their gender self-identity that defines them as transgender.

triad—a relationship between three people who choose to romantically and sexually engage with each other.

unicorn—a bisexual woman who is sought after by heterosexual couples in order to create a triad relationship. So-called because of their rarity in the wild.

unicorn hunter—a derogatory term for heterosexual couples seeking a third to add to their relationship, usually with little thought or care as to how to incorporate this third in a way that is ethical and respectful

vee—a relationship connection between three people, forming the shape of a V. One person in the "pivot" or "hinge" position is involved with two partners who are not romantically or sexually involved with each other.

veto—a specific relationship agreement or rule wherein one partner has the power to request that the other partner end one or all of their outside relationships

Notes

Intro

1. Fredrickson, Barbara. "Positivity Resonance and Loving-Kindness." Online Lecture, Positive Psychology from The University of North Carolina at Chapel Hill, Chapel Hill, NC. Accessed July 2, 2015, https://www.coursera.org/learn/positive-psychology/lecture/R9DoI/what-is-love.

Chapter 1

1. Kinsey Institute, "Prevalence of Homosexuality study." Last updated 2015. http://www.kinseyinstitute.org/research/ak-hhscale.html
2. Dan Savage, "Meet the Monogamish," *The Stranger*, January 4, 2012, http://www.thestranger.com/seattle/SavageLove?oid=11412386.
3. "Madonna-whore Complex," *Applied Social Psychology Blog* (blog), October 3, 2015, https://sites.psu.edu/aspsy/2015/10/03/madonna-whore-complex/.
4. S. A. McLeod, "Social Identity Theory," *Simply Psychology*, 2008. www.simplypsychology.org/social-identity-theory.html.
5. Charles Ramirez-Berg, *Latino Images in Film: Stereotypes, Subversion, Resistance* (University of Texas Press, 2009), 13–37.
6. Mormon.org. "Do Mormons practice polygamy?" Accessed December 10, 2015, https://www.mormon.org/faq/practice-of-polygamy.
7. Church of Jesus Christ of Latter-Day Saints, *The Doctrine and Covenants*, Section 132, verses 61–63, https://www.lds.org/scriptures/dc-testament/dc/132?lang=eng.
8. Rachel McRady, "Mo'Nique Clarifies Open Marriage to Sidney Hicks: 'It Was My Idea'," *US Weekly*, November 20, 2015, http://www.usmagazine.com/celebrity-news/news/monique-clarifies-open-marriage-to-sidney-hicks-it-was-my-idea-w158048.
9. Felicia R. Lee, "Luckily, There's Plenty of Her for Everybody," *The New York Times*, August 5, 2007, http://query.nytimes.com/gst/fullpage.html?res=9407E3D6103EF936A3575BC0A9619C8B63.
10. Dossie Easton and Janet Hardy, *The Ethical Slut: A Practical Guide to Polyamory, Open Relationships, and Other Adventures* (Celestial Arts; 2nd edition, 2009), ebook edition, 13.
11. Plato, *The Symposium*, Trans. Benjamin Jowett (Pearson, 1956).
12. Tikva Wolf, "Soulmates," *Kimchi Cuddles* (webcomic), 2013, http://kimchicuddles.com/post/51559238268/soulmates.
13. Melissa Melms, "12 Signs You're in a Serious, Committed, For-Real Relationship," *Glamour*, April 10, 2012, http://www.glamour.com/sex-love-life/blogs/smitten/2012/04/12-signs-youre-in-a-serious-com.
14. Beca Grimm, "24 Signs You're in a 'For Real' Relationship Because You're Clearly Way Past 'Just Dating' At This Point," *Bustle*, May 30, 2015, http://www.bustle.com/articles/86337-24-signs-youre-in-a-for-real-relationship-because-youre-clearly-way-past-just-dating-at.
15. Jeanette Winterson, *Why Be Happy When You Could Be Normal?* (Vintage, 2012).

Chapter 2

1. Kurt W. Alt, et al, "Twenty-Five Thousand-Year-Old Triple Burial From Dolnı Vestonice: An Ice-Age Family?," *American Journal of Physical Anthropology* 102 (1997), 123–131.
2. Simon Andreae, *Anatomy of Desire* (Little Brown Company, 1998).
3. Raymond S. Nickerson, "Confirmation Bias: A Ubiquitous Phenomenon in Many Guises," *Review of General Psychology* (1998), 175–177.
4. Richard F. Taflinger, "Human Reproduction," *Biological Basis of Sex Appeal*, 1996, http://public.wsu.edu/~taflinge/biosex2.html.
5. "Bonobo Behavior," *Bonobo Reproduction*, Univerisity of Wisconsin Department of Animal Sciences (blog), accessed December 20, 2015, http://www.ansci.wisc.edu/jjp1/ansci_repro/misc/project_websites_07/thur07/bonobo%20reproduction/behavior.html.
6. Corin Apicella, "New study of hunter-gatherers suggests social networks sparked evolution of cooperation," *Phys.org*, January 25, 2012, http://phys.org/news/2012–01-hunter-gatherers-social-networks-evolution-cooperation.html.
7. Hannah Devlin, "Early men and women were equal, say scientists," *The Guardian*, May 14, 2015, https://www.theguardian.com/science/2015/may/14/early-men-women-equal-scientists.
8. Simon Copland, "Equality and polyamory: why early humans weren't The Flintstones," *The Guardian*, May 19, 2015, http://www.theguardian.com/science/blog/2015/may/19/equality-and-polyamory-why-early-humans-werent-the-flintstones.
9. Benjamin Grant Purzycki, "Comparison of the Traditional and Contemporary Extended Family Units of the Hopi and Lakota (Sioux): A Study of the Deterioration of Kinship Structures and Functions," *Nebraska Anthropologist* (2004), Paper 68, http://digitalcommons.unl.edu/cgi/viewcontent.cgi?article=1067&context=nebanthro.
10. Marc C. Mees, "Teach Them the Moral Way of Living: The Meeting of Huron Sexuality and European Religion," *Loyola University New Orleans Student Historical Journal* (1997), http://www.loyno.edu/~history/journal/1997–8/Mees.html.
11. "Native American Marriage," *Native American Netroots* (blog), October 4, 2011, http://nativeamericannetroots.net/diary/1084.
12. *Handbook of North American Indians Volume 11,* eds. William C. Sturtevant, Raymond J. DeMallie (Government Printing Office, 2001), 535.
13. Kirsten Glaeser, "Till Death Us Do Part: The Evolution of Monogamy," *Oglethorpe Journal of Undergraduate Research* (2014), 16–24, http://digitalcommons.kennesaw.edu/cgi/viewcontent.cgi?article=1043&context=ojur.
14. Ibid.
15. Ibid.
16. Katie Sauvain, "Agriculture, Industry, and the Spiritual Realm: How Religion, Technology, and the Environment Interweave," *Swarthmore College Environmental Studies*, last updated January 25, 2006, http://fubini.swarthmore.edu/~ENVS2/S2006/ksauvai1/envssecondessay.html.
17. Charles Fourier, *Theory of Social Organization* (New York: C. P. Somerby, 1876), http://legacy.fordham.edu/halsall/mod/1820fourier.asp.
18. Steven Kreis, "The Utopian Socialists: Charles Fourier," *The History Guide: Lectures on Modern European Intellectual History*, last updated August 3, 2006, http://www.historyguide.org/intellect/lecture21a.html.
19. "Utopian Socialism," *Digital History* (2016), ID 3540, http://www.digitalhistory.uh.edu/disp_textbook.cfm?smtID=2&psid=3540.
20. Church of Jesus Christ of Latter-Day Saints, *The Doctrine and Covenants*, Section 132, verses 61–63, https://www.lds.org/scriptures/dc-testament/dc/132?lang=eng.

21. "Utopian Socialism," *Digital History* (2016), ID 3540, http://www.digitalhistory .uh.edu/disp_textbook.cfm?smtID=2&psid=3540.
22. Kathleen M. Hogan, "John Humphrey Noyes and the Oneida Perfectionists," *University of Virginia American Studies Hypertext Project* (1996), http://xroads.virginia.edu/ ~hyper/hns/cities/oneida.html.
23. "Utopian Socialism," *Digital History* (2016), ID 3540, http://www.digitalhistory .uh.edu/disp_textbook.cfm?smtID=2&psid=3540.
24. "The Oneida Story," *Oneida Ltd* (1994), http://www.oneida.com/aboutoneida/ the-oneida-story.
25. Libby Copeland, "Making Love and Trouble," *Slate*, March 12, 2012, http://www .slate.com/articles/double_x/doublex/2012/03/polyamory_and_its_surprisingly_ woman_friendly_roots_.html.
26. Ellen Wayland-Smith, *Oneida: From Free Love Utopia to the Well-Set Table* (Picador, 2016), 125.
27. Shellie Clark, "The Sexual Revolution of the Roaring Twenties: Practice or Perception?" (Brockport University, 2015), https://www.academia.edu/14095520/ The_Sexual_Revolution_of_the_Roaring_Twenties_Practice_or_Perception.
28. Douglas W. Orr, MD, "Psychoanalysis and the Bloomsbury Group," Clemson University Digital Press (2004), http://tigerprints.clemson.edu/cudp_mono/16/.
29. Ibid.
30. Ibid
31. Sam Alexander, "Lytton Strachey," *The Modernism Lab at Yale University* (wiki), 2010, https://modernism.research.yale.edu/wiki/index.php/Lytton_Strachey.
32. Susanna Rustin, "Boom Time for the Bloomsbury Group," *The Guardian*, June 5, 2015, https://www.theguardian.com/books/2015/jun/05/bloomsbury-booming-legacy -celebrate-virginia-woolf.
33. Patricia A. Klemans, "'Being Born a Woman': A New Look at Edna St. Vincent Millay," *Colby Quarterly*, March 1979, http://digitalcommons.colby.edu/cgi/viewcontent .cgi?article=2350&context=cg.
34. Elizabeth Majerus, "Edna St. Vincent Millay's Life," *Modern American Poetry*, last updated 2000, http://www.english.illinois.edu/maps/poets/m_r/millay/millay.htm.
35. Ibid.
36. Shannon Musset, "Simone de Beauvoir," *Internet Encyclopedia of Philosophy*, accessed December 21, 2015, http://www.iep.utm.edu/beauvoir/.
37. Louise Menand, "Stand By Your Man: The Strange Liaison of Sartre and Beauvoir," *The New Yorker*, September 26, 2005, http://www.newyorker.com/magazine/2005/09/26/ stand-by-your-man.
38. Ben Isenberg, "Wonder Woman Identity Revealed in Lepore Lecture," *Hamilton College News*, September 25, 2015, http://www.hamilton.edu/news/story/wonder -woman-revealed-in-lepore-lecture.
39. Terry Gross, Interview with Jill Lepore, *Fresh Air*, October 27, 2014, http://www .npr.org/2014/10/27/359078315/the-man-behind-wonder-woman-was-inspired-by -both-suffragists-and-centerfolds.
40. Allan C. Carlson, "The Myth of the Fifties," *Modern Age*, Winter-Spring 2011, https://home.isi.org/myth-fiftiesbremthe-permissive-society-america-1941%E2%80%931965em -alan-petigny.
41. Kinsey Institute, "Alfred Kinsey's 1948 and 1953 Studies," accessed December 22, 2015, http://www.indiana.edu/~kinsey/research/ak-data.html.
42. Kinsey Institute, "The Development and Publication of Sexual Behavior in the Human Male and Sexual Behavior in the Human Female: 'The Kinsey Reports' of 1948 and 1953,'" accessed December 22, 2015, http://www.indiana.edu/~kinsey/about/early -controversy.html.

43. Brenda Frink, "The Pill and the Marriage Revolution," *Gender News*, The Clayman Institute for Gender Research, September 29, 2011, http://gender.stanford.edu/news/2011/pill-and-marriage-revolution.

44. Mindy Shalayne Popplewell, "Women in the Lifestyle: A Qualitative Look at the Perceptions, Attitudes, and Experiences of Women Who Swing," (Master's thesis, Western Kentucky University, December 2006), http://digitalcommons.wku.edu/cgi/viewcontent.cgi?article=1260&context=theses.

45. Melodee Lynn Sova, "Who Knows Their Bedroom Secrets? Communication Privacy Management in Couples Who Swing," (Master's thesis, University of North Texas, August 2012), http://digital.library.unt.edu/ark:/67531/metadc149665/m2/1/high_res_d/thesis.pdf.

46. Nena O'Neill and George O'Neill, "Open Marriage: A Synergic Model," *The Family Coordinator*, 21 (Oct 1972), 403-409.

47. "Timeline of the Kerista Commune," Kerista Commune, accessed December 23, 2015, http://www.kerista.com/timeline.html.

48. Lawrence Hamelin, "And to No More Settle for Less Than Purity: Reflections on the Kerista Commune," *University of Colorado at Denver Journal*, August 2013, https://www.academia.edu/4897458/And_To_No_More_Settle_For_Less_Than_Purity_Reflections_on_the_Kerista_Commune.

49. Ibid.

50. Prudence Jones, "What is Paganism?" *PaganFederation.org*, accessed June 24, 2016. http://www.paganfederation.org/what-is-paganism/.

51. Christine Hoff Kraemer, "Gender and Sexuality in Contemporary Paganism," *Religious Compass* (Blackwell Publishing 2012), 6/8, 390–401, https://www.academia.edu/2286523/Gender_and_Sexuality_in_Contemporary_Paganism.

52. Daniel Cardoso, "Polyamory, or The Harshness of Spawning a Substantive Meme," *Interact*, 2011 (17), https://www.academia.edu/592878/Polyamory_or_The_Harshness_of_Spawning_a_Substantive_Meme.

53. Alan M., Loving More, "History of Loving More," accessed December 26, 2015, http://www.lovemore.com/aboutus/history/.

54. Deborah Anapol, *Love Without Limits: The Quest for Sustainable Intimate Relationships* (IntiNet Resource Center, 1992).

55. Alan M., Loving More, "History of Loving More," accessed December 26, 2015, http://www.lovemore.com/aboutus/history/.

56. Cuddle Party, "About Us." accessed December 27, 2015, http://www.cuddleparty.com.

57. Brenden Shucart, "Polyamory by the Numbers," *The Advocate*, January 8, 2016, http://www.advocate.com/current-issue/2016/1/08/polyamory-numbers.

Chapter 3

1. Off the Relationship Escalator, "What is the Relationship Escalator?" Accessed June 23, 2016, http://offescalator.com/what-escalator/.

Chapter 4

1. Klean Radio, Interview with Dr. Pat Allen, February 17, 2015, http://www.kleanradio.com/2015/02/17/talking-sex-love-addiction-dr-pat-allen/.

2. United Farm Workers. "History of Sí Se Puede," accessed June 26, 2016, http://www.ufw.org/_board.php?mode=view&b_code=cc_his_research&b_no=5970.

3. "Sí Se Puede," *Wikipedia*, last updated June 9, 2016, https://en.wikipedia.org/wiki/S%C3%AD_se_puede.

4. Michael P. Carey, PhD and Andrew D. Forsyth, "Teaching Tip Sheet: Self-Efficacy," American Psychological Association, accessed January 2, 2016. http://www.apa.org/pi/aids/resources/education/self-efficacy.aspx.
5. Multiamory, Interview with Franklin Veaux, July 15, 2015, http://www.multiamory .com/podcast/27-franklin-veaux-and-eve-rickert.
6. Jessica Graham, email to the author, June 30, 2015.

Chapter 5

1. Stephen M. Garcia, Avishalom Tor, and Tyrone M. Schiff, "The Psychology of Competition: A Social Comparison Perspective," *Perspectives on Psychological Science*, 2013, 8(6) 634–650, http://www-personal.umich.edu/~smgarcia/pubs/psych%20of%20competition.pdf.
2. Ibid.
3. Lissa Rankin, "Permission to Break My Heart," *Lissa Rankin, MD* (blog), July 31, 2011, http://lissarankin.com/permission-to-break-my-heart.
4. Sophie Curtis, "Men Twice as Likely to 'Mobile Snoop' than Women," *The Telegraph*, September 10, 2013, http://www.telegraph.co.uk/technology/news/10298731/Men-twice-as-likely-to-mobile-snoop-than-women.html.
5. Dossie Easton and Janet Hardy, *The Ethical Slut: A Practical Guide to Polyamory, Open Relationships, and Other Adventures* (Celestial Arts; 2nd edition, 2009), ebook edition, 56.
6. Jennice Vilhauer, Ph.D, "What to Do When You Can't Stop Thinking About Something," *Psychology Today*, December 30, 2015, https://www.psychologytoday.com/blog/living-forward/201512/what-do-when-you-cant-stop-thinking-about-it.

Chapter 6

1. Jessica Graham, instant message to author, March 18, 2016.
2. Alanna Vagianos, "This Is How Often Women Masturbate," *The Huffington Post*, August 12, 2014, http://www.huffingtonpost.com/2014/06/04/women-masturbation -statistics-fivethirtyeight_n_5445530.html.
3. Heather A. Rupp, Ph.D, and Kim Wallen, Ph.D, "Sex Differences in Response to Visual Sexual Stimuli: A Review," *Arch Sex Behavioral Journal*, August 1, 2007, 37(2) 206–218, http://www.ncbi.nlm.nih.gov/pmc/articles/PMC2739403/.
4. Jim Dryden, "Erotic images elicit strong response from brain," *Washington University in St. Louis Newsroom*, June 8, 2006, http://news.wustl.edu/news/Pages/7319.aspx.
5. The Asexuality Visibility & Education Network, "About Asexuality," accessed March 23, 2015, http://www.asexuality.org/home/?q=overview.html.
6. Ibid.
7. UC Berkeley Gender Equity Resource Center, "LGBT Definition of Terms," accessed June 28, 2016, http://geneq.berkeley.edu/lgbt_resources_definiton_of_terms.
8. Demisexuality Resource Center, "What is Demisexuality?," accessed June 23, 2016, http://demisexuality.org/articles/what-is-demisexuality/.
9. Ibid.
10. Martin P. Kafka, "Hypersexual Disorder: A Proposed Diagnosis for the DSM-V," American Psychiatric Association (2009), http://www.dsm5.org/Research/Documents/Kafka_Hypersexual_ASB.pdf.
11. Ibid.

Chapter 7

1. Kathy Labriola, "Models of Open Relationships," *The Lesbian Polyamory Reader* (Haworth Press, 1999), http://socrates.bmcc.cuny.edu/jbisz/websiteBB/Models_of_Open_Relationships_01/ModelsofOpenRelationships.pdf.
2. Andie Nordgren, "The Short Instructional Manifesto for Relationship Anarchy," *Andie's Log* (blog), July 6, 2012, http://log.andie.se/.
3. Aesop, "The Oak and the Reeds," *Aesop's Fables*, accessed July 2, 2015, http://www.aesopfables.com/cgi/aesop1.cgi?3&TheOakandtheReeds.

Chapter 8

1. Nirmala, *Gifts with No Giver: A Love Affair with Truth* (CreateSpace Independent Publishing Platform, 2008).
2. Markus Schlosser, "Agency," *Stanford Encyclopedia of Philosophy*, 2015, http://plato.stanford.edu/entries/agency/.
3. Ralph Waldo Emerson, "Give All to Love," *English poetry III: from Tennyson to Whitman.*, ed. Charles W. Eliot (P.F. Collier & Son, 1914).
4. Love Is Respect, "Is This Abuse?" accessed May 13, 2016, http://www.loveisrespect.org/is-this-abuse/types-of-abuse/.

Chapter 9

1. Brenden Shucart, "Polyamory by the Numbers," *The Advocate*, January 8, 2016, http://www.advocate.com/current-issue/2016/1/08/polyamory-numbers.

Chapter 10

1. Dr. Elisabeth Sheff, *The Polyamorists Next Door: Inside Multiple-Partner Relationships and Families* (Rowman & Littlefield Publishers, 2013).

Chapter 11

1. Neela Ghoshal and Kyle Knight, "Rights in Transition: Making Legal Recognition for Transgender People a Global Priority," Human Rights Watch World Report 2016, accessed November 8, 2016, https://www.hrw.org/world-report/2016/rights-in-transition.
2. UN Women, "Facts and figures: Leadership and political participation." Last updated August 2016, http://www.unwomen.org/en/what-we-do/leadership-and-political-participation/facts-and-figures.
3. Alison Symington, Intersectionality: A Tool for Gender and Economic Justice, Association for Women's Rights in Development, 2004. https://lgbtq.unc.edu/sites/lgbtq.unc.edu/files/documents/intersectionality_en.pdf.
4. Dr. Elisabeth Sheff, "The Polyamorous Possibility and Fear of the OTHER," *elisabethsheff* (blog), September 12, 2013, https://elisabethsheff.com/2013/09/12/the-polyamorous-possibility-and-fear-of-the-other/.
5. Elisabeth Sheff, email to the author, May 9, 2016.
6. "In re M.C.," *Justia US Law*, accessed June 23, 2016, http://law.justia.com/cases/california/court-of-appeal/2011/b222241/.
7. Brenden Shucart, "Polyamory by the Numbers," *The Advocate*, January 8, 2016, http://www.advocate.com/current-issue/2016/1/08/polyamory-numbers.
8. Ibid.
9. Pepper Mint, "Non-monogamy for Men: The Big Picture," *freaksexual* (blog), November 5, 2009, https://freaksexual.com/2009/11/05/non-monogamy-for-men-the-big-picture/.

INDEX